Foodergies!
Eat Right with Food Families

LAURA KEILES, ND

DISCLAIMER: The medical statements or information provided in this literature must be considered an educational service only. It is recommended that this information is used in conjunction with a visit with qualified health care professionals.

No action by the reader should be taken based solely on the contents of this book. The natural treatments and suggestions discussed here, can affect different people in different ways, occasionally producing adverse reactions. Readers who fail to consult appropriate health authorities assume the risk of any injuries.

Because of the constant changes resulting from ongoing research and clinical experience, some of the literature presented may not be current. The author and publisher are not responsible for errors and/or omissions.

The purpose is to provide you with the information that will educate you to make more educated health and dietary decisions as applicable.

ISBN: 0-9884624-0-0
ISBN-13: 979-0-9884624-0-3

DEDICATION

To my "sisters" who inspired me and cheered me on through numerous food changes before I found my food groove.

To my husband - Doug and my sons – Jordan and Matthew, who have gotten used to and embraced the gluten free, dairy free, tree nut free, soy free, nightshade free Mom and continue to help her stay pain free.

CONTENTS

ACKNOWLEDGMENTS   i

1 INTRODUCTION   1

2 ALLERGIES, SENSITIVITIES, AND INTOLERANCES, OH MY   7

3 LET'S GET STARTED   25

4 GRASSES & GRAINS   48

5 ANIMAL PROTEINS & DAIRY   61

6 LEGUMES   82

7 NIGHTSHADES   88

8 NUTS & SEEDS   96

9 FUNGI   118

10 COMMONLY CONSUMED FRUIT & VEGETABLES   125

11 SUPPORTING DOCUMENTS & LINKS   165

GLOSSARY   167

BIBLIOGRAPHY   177

ONLINE REFERENCES   184

INDEX   194

ABOUT THE AUTHOR   205

ACKNOWLEDGMENTS

This book is the fruit of a seven year journey to solve the riddles of my own health issues and digestive distress. Much of that time it was not clear that my research would lead to a book to educate others to find their own answers. While I looked for information, I earned a living as a Software Delivery Architect and Project Management consultant and went to school part time to gain a Doctorate of Naturopathy degree. Now looking back on all I have accomplished, I wonder how I juggled it all, along with a husband and two kids. Those who know me are not surprised at all. The work paid off; I absorbed and applied all I learned and lost 40 pounds and regained my health. The process has been challenging and frustrating, causing me to rethink the most basic element of all our lives: the food we eat. In the end, this journey has been my great reward for what I learned and for those who taught and inspired and supported me along the way. I hope you find answers in these pages and benefit from my years of research.

The traditional medical community at large has not always been the most effective, at finding what the source of my health issues was. I was always "within normal limits" from a standard blood test perspective. On occasion I would exhibit a slightly high glucose or cholesterol level when I was not taking care of myself. It was always within statistical range so why worry? I did because in my heart I knew it was not right. I was not healthy regardless off what my data stated. The few detail oriented physicians, who think and process patterns and trends in information like I do, helped me make a difference in my health.

Personal instincts and detailed research paved the way for this work. I write this in honor of my key educational role models – Dr. Elson Haas, Dr. Michael Greer, Dr. Joel Fuhrman, Dr. John Douillard, Dr. Christiane Northrup and Dr. Mark Hyman. These brilliant physicians teach that we are bio-individuals, electro-chemical machines. Their work demonstrates that food can be supportive or subversive to the efficiency of the machine – which is us. You *really* are what you eat; and what you become is a direct result of what you eat. I did not want to keep feeding myself toxins directly or indirectly any longer. I also wanted to make sure others were informed enough so they could do the same.

I would also like to thank Dr. Peter Osborne and Sayer Ji for their investigational diligence through Glutenology and GreenMedInfo.com in making my research to support this book easier. Being a data geek for most of my life and watching the internet flourish – both information and misinformation are now widely available. It is important to decipher the best scientific and anecdotal studies and statistics to confirm and validate the information shared. There were a plethora of entries to choose from and years of digging and reviewing articles and books finally showed consensus and consistency in the message I was trying to convey.

Immense thanks to Karen Wright, Traditional ND, Health Coach and CNHP for her technical review of this work and keeping me accurate and properly referenced. Thanks to Gerald Linn, Susan Knopf, Alexz Rosen, Sherry Wheaton and others for the K-I-S-S review as a laypersons and health nuts for making sure that I did not go too far on the jargon. A special acknowledgement goes to the co-creator of the term "Foodergies", Jason Perlow. This term evolved during the discussion of foods eaten, allergic and sensitive and how we could describe that behavior simply.

I have been blessed to have my family be a part of this journey and still want to be around after all the psychological, physical and dietary tumult. They witnessed my shifts, my eliminations, my proactive and reactive therapies as well as my successes and failures. They have provided their unwavering support in the crafting of this work. The completion of this effort has been one of the key defining moments in my life.

I have finally achieved my own personal quality compliance – I set my goal to get healthy and remove my pain. I did it through planned diet and lifestyle changes. I proved it by being able to repeat the process and maintain my health; my project management buddies know what I mean. Lastly, I heartily thank my many friends and colleagues as they have gotten used to "what I do eat" versus "what I don't eat" and think that way for others as well. It is an honor to share this effort with you.

Wishing you abundant health –

Laura Keiles
PMP, ND, HC, AADP
January 2013

.

1 INTRODUCTION

When I told my friends and colleagues that I was writing a book based on my health journey, there was no surprise. They always wanted me to write down my recipes for the crazy food combinations I would come up with and I said that would be in another book. First I wanted to tell the story and explain my plan around identifying food intolerances through food families. I didn't want this book to be just like any other food information or diet or nutritional guidance. I have been wrestling with my own nutritional deficiencies and health for the last five years. This book is the culmination of my personal research and experience with my clients as a Naturopath.

In May 2005 it became clear to me that modern medicine did not have all the answers. I had been attempting to function with postpartum depression for the two years prior, and was at the end of my rope health-wise. I would wake up more tired than I went to bed – sleep was not restorative. I was not hungry, though I made sure to eat decently. I would have blackouts and dizzy spells - while sitting on the floor next to my kids, while commuting at the train station and collapsing for a few seconds and once behind the wheel of the car. At that point, I went to seek more help. The specialists in neurology, endocrinology, cardiology and hematology had no answers. I am a person who likes to have reasonable, logical answers or else I get edgy, angry, especially when it comes to my health or my family's. I went to a psychiatrist to see if it was really all in my head and to talk to someone instead of being obsessively cranky because I wanted an answer that no physician could give. That psychiatrist figured it out, that it was not in my head, directly that is. Post partum depression is a tricky thing, especially the bout I was going through. He prescribed "commercial medicine" and it stopped the spells. The medicine worked for awhile, then the side effects of weight gain and tremors kicked in and new medicine was prescribed for the side effects; that was the last straw. As an amateur homeopath since 1995 I figured it was time to put all the "new-which-is-really-old" concepts into play in my life on a consistent basis. I found a Naturopath to help me deal with my postpartum depression along with my diet, and started using homeopathic versions of the commercial medicine. There was improvement, no more tremors or side effects and yet not everything he recommended worked to keep me consistently stable and in better health. So I was back to the "me" who was normal as per doctors. It was just not the "me" I wanted and needed to be.

I have always been a researcher at heart. Data mining/analytics was my day job, so why not learn how to heal myself on my terms? It is just more data and processing, which comes naturally to me. So, I went back to school and studied to become a Naturopath. I needed to learn what was necessary to know to heal myself. I have always had "the need to know" gene – as I would not always accept the first answer given due to my very quizzical nature, I would review it and look for additional fact/data/detail to support the claim. Also, isn't the mantra of most good doctors is "Doctor, heal thyself first"? I started that journey. I made changes to my diet, reduced my sugars, cut back on the white food products and yet I only made minimal headway. I had not researched or investigated enough - something was missing. I had absorbed every piece of knowledge I could from my studies and applied it as often as I could to my own life. It took a meeting through an online seminar during school with Dr. Elson Haas that I could say changed my life as I know it. Dr. Haas pioneered eating with the seasons as well as staying healthy with nutrition through the seasons as much as John Douillard did. He also supported the concept of cleansing annually and not only juice cleanses or fasts like many doctors such as Dr. Joel Fuhrman purport. I respect all these practitioners as they were instrumental as sources of input and knowledge that allowed me to come to this point today.

The concept of food sensitivities and intolerances were new to me back then and to reduce and eliminate them became my mantra. From May 2009 forward it became more and more evident that the foods I ate led to toxins in my body that I could not get rid of. Dr. Haas called it "False Fat" and for me it really was. When I stopped eating those foods that had those toxins my body could not process or deal with, my body started to heal itself slowly and steadily. I would say that after the first year and a half I made major headway. I had lost 25 pounds; I knew my end-weight and health goal which was now in sight. Above all I wanted to be pain free. I had found out in April 2008 that I had arthritis, and needed to be closer to my best weight and health for my build to help alleviate it. I kept a specific practice in mind; I decided to take it slow and analyze everything I ate. In fact, I have consistently kept a daily food journal since January 2010. That's a long time to be tracking your food. What I discovered through tracking my food was how I felt by eating specific foods but also how it impacted the amount of physical pain stiffness and joints or digestive upset I had. I tracked it all and I saw patterns in the data collected. You cannot take the data geek out of me and so I kept reviewing my journal to find my answers.

There are those who would say it was me losing the weight that made the pain go away – well, the pain was still there, and in fact worse at times. Even with exercise and physical therapy with a lower weight or not, the pain was debilitating. There are those who said I was going to waste away and make myself deficient on what little I was eating – not so because there was still plenty things I could eat. Others said it was a lot of woo-hoo, witch doctor stuff I would be learning as a Naturopath. That statement amuses me because the earliest Naturopaths were scientists, osteopaths and homeopaths who did what I did – heal themselves. Each of the great Naturopaths (Benedict Lust, Arnold Rikli, and Henry Lindlahr to name a few) were people who themselves worked to find cures to their own ailments through the traditional health means of their time. Those early Naturopaths went back to the beginnings of health – nature and the elements. Practitioners back in the time of those men could not help their patients be asymptomatic or truly cure someone – they could just cover the symptoms until they went away on their own or got new ones to tackle and the others were no longer urgent anymore. There is an old adage which says "Those who do not know the history are condemned to repeat it" – it is no different in the advent of medicine in the last century. The more "science" that is applied to what the early medicine men, herbal healers and shamans knew the more modern science is finding the "why" behind it. The only issue is that we have lost a lot of this traditional knowledge, experience, and documentation. Yes, those things help science be more accurate and astute and one of those things that integrative health practitioners (MDs) and naturopaths agree on is that "Food can be medicine or toxin". However, which one is *your* medicine or toxin remains to be determined.

I felt like a modern day Samuel Hahnemann (father of Homeopathy) – a dietary and homeopathic guinea pig - I questioned everything that I knew, tried new foods and eliminated others to make me better. I embraced the fact that I was an impatient person, exposed and raised in a microwave society. I had to learn that everything has its time. I knew that I would not be feeding and adding to my arthritis in this new way of life/eating. However living with the pain and travel abuse of my day job, it was time to get clean and get healed once and for all. I find it troublesome that a mid-40 year old woman had 75+ year old arthritis. Could it have been my extra 20-40 lbs for 13 years? – No, as per my Family Doctor and Orthopedist; it was a mystery to both of them. Could it have been restricted movement cutting off blood flow and allowing calcium deposits to appear? Not likely – though it had a small potential. Were genetics a factor? Sure, there was arthritis in my family history – just not this early in life. Were the years of travel abuse a factor? – Somewhat, except that would show more wear and tear not calcium deposits and bone spurs. Again, no answers that made sense for "why" could be found.

I had to have shoulder surgery to remove the bone spurs so that I could work and travel as an IT Professional. It was a matter of necessity. A recent review of my shoulder surgery from 2 years ago showed that no calcium deposits or arthritic areas have come back. In fact there is no sign of inflammation in that area either. Why is that? My lifestyle is different and my diet is different. The answer to the question of HOW I got arthritis still eluded me. My orthopedic surgeon recommended the rheumatologist I currently see today. She is all about the scientific approach in problem solving. She does not belittle my approach to data collection or analysis. In fact she assimilated it, added it to hers and together we are pinning down the answers. Together we have surmised that part of the cause was my recent discovery of having the gene for Celiac Disease. Also there is the perspective of issues with Nightshades and Vitamin D deficiency from years of being an indoors computer geek. Over 3 years ago, I went through a dietary elimination challenge-response diet. This specific elimination/challenge was planned using all the knowledge and research done during my studies. From that analysis I had determined that gluten, soy, nightshade plants and dairy were the most likely culprits and eliminated them before even working with her. So when informed of the genetic situation she stated amusingly with a smile, "Gee, I don't have to tell you to be gluten free, you already knew to do that." The official verdict is still out on the Nightshades-Vitamin D correlation (which there is one) and we are still analyzing to confirm.

There is nothing wrong with being an informed patient, though my perspective is as opinionated as the physicians. One cannot debate statements of fact that are in concert with the standard education of a physician. So then they have to think harder and do their job more – just like science intends the medical community at large to do, and share it. Does this sound hokey to you anymore?

You want your life to be more than a number; you want to make a difference – to have an impact. These things are important to everyone (well most folks for sure), not just a Naturopath or certified Project Management Professional. I am no different than you, dear reader, looking for answers and especially when I needed to look inside myself for some of them and not the world outside of me. I continued to be in pain because my spirit was in pain – stifled, caged and restricted – just like my arms and shoulders positioned to type and work a mouse or to drag and lift multiple computers around in an airport and sleep away from my home.

I went to back to school to learn, to heal and to help others with their health through education and coaching. I want to make a difference in both worlds, perhaps I did not see that I did and maybe I did not want to see the negative lessons I was learning. I would rather learn positive lessons. Regardless I am grateful and thankful for both types of lessons. It is the balance of things. With all the education and experiences, it was last year when I discovered the intuitive gift of walking a labyrinth. Studies have shown its brain balancing properties – how it equalizes neurological pathways and provides focus and smooth thought processing. The experience I had, in the labyrinth at Kripalu Institute in Stockbridge, Massachusetts, guided me here now, to share this message with you.

The essence of the message for this book is thus – food family identification is **crucial** in the investigation of our health. Personally, I am working a more seasonal diet, intermingled with detoxification cleanses and sticking to those food families that work for me to remove the last of my positive autoimmune signature and reverse my arthritis and keep Celiac disease at bay once and for all. To assist me in achieving my goals, I am a member of an organic community garden. I have three plots of 15 ft by 15 ft to grow foods and flowers in a harmonious setting, among other like minded health conscious gardeners. This outdoor activity serves many purposes. It allows me to connect with and be educated by nature directly in how things grow and mature. Communing with other gardeners also helps me find the best foods to grow based on our region, for me, my family and friends. Besides that, I get some desperately needed outdoor time to obtain some Vitamin D naturally.

I have been looking for this kind of information that I am documenting for you for over 3 years. It has been a labor of love and has become the guidelines for my educating others on how to find what works for them. This is the same detail I used in my research for myself - how to break it down so I could be more discreet with my food family choices. It did not exist in a form like this, scattered through out the internet and in pieces and clips as simplified level in books. I am pleased to present this to you for your education and reference.

Finding foods that are your friends and not your foes is not a walk in a labyrinth – it is like a maze. I hope you find the information in this book helpful, to guide you through your own food family maze. Find those food-allergies/sensitivities, "Foodergies™" as I call them, and have it be a simple course of what stays in and what comes out of your daily consumption. Once on that path, it becomes the journey to improve your health.

2 ALLERGIES, SENSITIVITIES, AND INTOLERANCES, OH MY

Let's take a moment to discuss the finer points of allergies, sensitivities and intolerances. I like to call them Foodergies™ – the meshing of food and its impact on your health. For some, it is not an issue and I am thankful to hear that. For others, living with allergies, sensitivities and intolerances is no picnic, and I can completely relate to them.

For example, I used to eat bell peppers frequently when I was younger; they were often my snack in the afternoon. One day in my teens, I started to get more digestive upset and heartburn – so I stopped eating them exclusively. I still ate potatoes, hot peppers and tomatoes a lot. Through my recent dietary evaluations, I found out that not eating them relieved some if not most of my arthritic pain. Why is that? The plant family that potatoes, tomatoes, hot peppers and bell peppers share is called Solanaceae - Nightshades. Members of that plant family have two toxic compounds glycoalkaloid (poisons) in them which can trigger an immune response and produce calcification and pain – *calcitriol* and *solanine*; so what would that be called – a sensitivity or an intolerance?

Using that example – let's investigate deeper what happens in the body. A member of the Solanaceae family – green bell pepper – is consumed raw. When we chew we release enzymes in our saliva to break this plant down. For some people, there is an insufficiency of digestive enzymes in the saliva and stomach which can lead to gastric upset. Over time our digestive system can be depleted through the things we eat requiring a retraining or a supplementation to make it be more efficient again. Depending on age, current state of health and genetic disposition, retraining may take longer to perform. Temporary supportive supplementation of enzymes is a good choice while the engine gets a dietary tune up.

Once the plant has made it to the stomach to be broken down into chyme, the next place is in the digestive pathways where the immune responses come into play. The pancreas juices get released neutralizing the acidic chyme from the stomach. Those juices contain the key enzymes necessary to break down the plant sugars into a better digested form in the small intestine. The small intestine is responsible for absorbing nutrients and passing them into the bloodstream. Whatever is left is passed through to the large intestine to be processed and then excreted out of the body.

The small intestine may have been compromised from other dietary issues – the villi are flattened and not able to do the filtering and allow potential toxins to pass into the bloodstream along with any nutrients. The commonly used term for that is "leaky gut". This compromised intestinal condition short circuits the chemical engine's processing. So depending on the immune reaction, members of the family Solanaceae can produce both sensitivity and intolerance.

Immunity

There were two key articles in support of this book that I reviewed with respect to food sensitivities and allergies from Dr. Peter Osborne of the Gluten Free Society – glutenfreesociety.org: "*Doctor Denial: Why Most Doctors Ignore Gluten Sensitivity*" and "*Why are some Doctors scarred of Gluten Sensitivity?*". I agree with the perception by the medical community at large; when folks describe their experiences and are not clearly able to articulate what is going on in their bodies, they are dismissed. Have you ever been told you can't be allergic to 'X' because your skin test or RAST test says you're not? I have been there and done that personally. Ok – you may not have an "allergy" in conventional terms. It may be considered an intolerance or sensitivity. In fact, the food sensitive or allergic population rates have doubled in the last 20 years and the severity of those reactions has increased as well. What most people attribute allergy to is called an IgE (Immunoglobulin Type E) reaction. This reaction is the result of the antibody that is produced which reacts to a food or airborne inhalants.

There is a chain of reactions in the body which release histamine into the bloodstream. The resulting reaction shows in the skin as itching or hives, or through respiratory distress, congestion, and digestive distress or in worst-case significant swelling to the point of suffocation (anaphylaxis). There are many lab tests that will diagnose a true food allergy. The most common food allergies which are dangerous surround the following food families: legumes (soy and peanuts), tree nuts, shellfish, dairy and wheat products (and their members).

So do people really have food allergies or are there more intolerances? Well, they can have both. Food intolerance or sensitivities involve the immune system response which may or may not be coupled with the IgE allergic histamine response. The other immune system responses – IgA, IgG, IgD and IgM are slower to respond and surface in the body. Those immune responses share similar symptoms as digestive distress, congestive issues as well as skin eruptions. Food intolerance may also be a result of a deficiency, for example missing the lactase enzyme in one's digestive tract shows up as lactose intolerance. So, if the body has digestive issues, then there may be a compromised immune system. If that is the case, then the immune system responses may end up being more prevalent and as a result, ill health exists.

The five general categories of antibody reactions – IgE, IgA, IgD, IgG, and IgM – describe how the body reacts to something invading our bodies. The invasion can come from some sort of pathogen or something we inhale, breaks in our skin, and/or the consuming of food. We do have some initial defenses like the tonsils, adenoids, the cilia in our nasal passages and the stomach acid which deter most of them.

   ❧ IgE – This is the type of reaction that is considered acute and truly an allergy - especially in the deadly allergies that is well known in the news – peanuts, nuts, and crustaceans especially. It is the antibody that allergist tests for when they perform the skin prick allergy assessments. This antibody facilitates the release of histamines and other chemicals which fight large invaders such as parasites. The IgE is fairly sensitive and can also respond to harmless allergens, just as it would a parasite, resulting in the typical allergic symptoms.

What if what you ate was an issue, though it did not produce an immediate response? There are four other antibodies which handle those types of reactions. The other antibody reactions are types of delayed hypersensitivities:

- ∾ IgA – Occurs mainly in fluid such as saliva, tears, breast milk and digestive juices. It is also the first line of defense against airborne antigens coming through the mucosal areas before they enter the bloodstream.

- ∾ IgD – Occurs on the outer membranes of the B cells. It helps identify foreign antigens. It is part of the immunity structure which helps immune responses switch between one class of antibody to another.

- ∾ IgG – This is a wide ranging antibody found through out the organs and blood vessels. This is the specific antibody which can be used to identify most of the food sensitivities and intolerances. These antibodies have a longer life span than the other antibodies. The degree and severity of symptoms expressed from an IgG reaction can vary due to bioindividuality and the amount of the offending food ingested. These antibodies are created due to a large/length exposure to a food antigen. Instead of binding to the mast cells like in a IgE response – the antibody binds to the food itself, creating immune complexes. The more of these immune complexes that there are, the more your immune system is activated and it gradually builds up bringing your system into full tilt reaction similar to an IgE. That is why it can take a few hours to days, or even weeks to show up. IgG is produced after the first line IgM antibody has started to clean up invading antigens; essentially when the immune system has established that the antigen is a real threat to the body. IgG hangs around to "maintain the immunity defenses" to make sure the same antigen is incapable of causing disease or reaction a second time. It is the same immune response that occurs after a vaccination to defend the body against the virus/bacteria found in the vaccine.

  ⅋ IgM – is so large it stays inside the blood vessels and seeks out antigens and mops up many antigens at a time - it is the first line of immunological defense against foreign molecules in the bloodstream.

Let's look at the symptomatic similarities and differences between antibody reactions as documented by Dr. Jonathan Brostoff in *Food allergies and food intolerance: the complete guide to their identification and treatment:*

Symptom	Food Allergy (IgE, IgA)	Intolerance/ Sensitivity (IgM,IgG)
Hives	Often	Rarely
Airway Constriction	Often	Rarely
Asthma	Often	Rarely
Wheezing	Often	Rarely
Itching	Often	Rarely
Drop in blood pressure	Often	Rarely
Shock	Sometimes	Rarely
Weak Pulse	Sometimes	Rarely
Rapid Pulse	Sometimes	Sometimes
Dizziness	Sometimes	Sometimes
Watery eyes	Often	Sometimes
Runny nose	Often	Sometimes
Skin rash	Often	Sometimes
Skin eruptions	Sometimes	Sometimes
Swollen tongue	Sometimes	Rarely
Irritable bowels	Rarely	Often
Abdominal cramping	Often	Often
Vomiting	Often	Often
Diarrhea	Often	Often
Nausea	Often	Often
Fainting	Sometimes	Rarely
Itchy mouth	Often	Rarely
Lightheadedness	Sometimes	Sometimes
Drooling	Sometimes	Rarely
Inability to swallow	Sometimes	Rarely
Change in voice quality	Sometimes	Rarely

Redness	Often	Sometimes
Fever or warmth (flushing)	Often	Sometimes
Bladder infections	Rarely	Sometimes
Ear infections	Sometimes	Sometimes
Joint pain	Rarely	Sometimes
Low back pain	Rarely	Sometimes
Migraine	Rarely	Sometimes
Headache non migraine	Sometimes	Sometimes
Sinusitis	Often	Often
Itchy throat	Often	Rarely
Sore throat	Sometimes	Often
Constipation	Rarely	Sometimes
Gastritis	Rarely	Sometimes
Ulcers	Rarely	Sometimes
Depression	Rarely	Sometimes
Anxiety	Sometimes	Sometimes
Chronic fatigue	Rarely	Sometimes
Panic attacks	Sometimes	Sometimes

These four antibody reactions are specifically used by medical practitioners in the identification food sensitivities, intolerances and non IgE allergies. During my evaluation of food families over 3 years ago, I performed dietary elimination and corresponding challenge tests against glutens and other sensitive foods, and determined which one of those foods did not work for me. Recently, I found out I possessed one of the two primary Celiac Disease genes (HLA-DQ8) through testing with my Rheumatologist. She stated, since I was already functioning on a gluten free level, she did not have to instruct me to eliminate it. This is a case of listening to ones' body and documenting reactions being completely accurate. I received confirmation that everything I had been doing, observing and tracking were spot on.

Celiac Disease can be the result of an untreated Gluten Sensitivity as well as genetic – so it is like the Chicken and the egg for me. Did I actually have Celiac Disease even when the tests came back negative / normal for IgE Wheat/Gluten? Or what sensitivity has gone too far enabled by my genes? Either way, my gut was not happy and my diet had to change for me to start my healing.

Also, due to our compromised immune systems – the inability to produce enough B cells to keep the intolerances and allergies at bay – gluten/wheat and dairy have been seen to be as debilitating in our young children. Notice the coincidental rise in autism spectrum and attention deficit disorder. What has happened to us? Since when was it that the food we ate or were exposed to is one of the sources of our compromised immunity? Look at the rise in nut allergy and peanut allergies since I was a child (over 40 years ago). I can remember a single person – one – when I was growing up who had a deathly reaction to peanuts. We were also told that they had many food allergies too, and that person's health was always in question. I was one who had allergies too, which were nut based and considered more common an anaphylaxis reaction and reasonable where allergies were concerned. To have odd food allergies was a stigma of compromised health and poor genetics. I am saddened by the increased need for inhalers due to asthma, or epi-pens to prevent death due to accidental exposure to those toxins, among other allergens.

Detoxification and Cleanses

During my time of pain and stress, I had already started to cut back on carbohydrates, eat more vegetables, juice more, and even exercise. I still did not feel entirely better. I still had aches and pains, my weight had not changed much at all even with eating less - nothing budged. As mentioned earlier one of the online seminars from my Naturopathy school was with Dr. Elson Haas - author of the books *Staying Healthy with Nutrition*, *The False Fat Diet* and *The New Detox Diet*. Our primary reading for the class was *Staying Healthy with Nutrition* and from that he had recommended performing detox annually. Early in Dr. Haas' practice one of his patients called him out for being overweight and a smoker. The patient did not find the him to be a role model being in that condition and that left a severe impact on Dr. Haas. That lesson he shared stuck with me - it truly was Doctor heal thyself, and that's just what Dr. Elson did; and here he was teaching future naturopaths the same lesson. So I took that lesson a step further. I went on to read *The Detox Diet* and *The False Fat Diet*, that he had written, and the bells went off in my head. What struck me as important was that although doing a cleanse properly was crucial to cleaning out any toxins, it was the time *after* the cleanse which actually made the biggest impact on my health.

All benefits of the cleanse are reversed if you go back to the way you used to eat afterwards. I wasn't going to let that happen. I kept a diary of the foods I ate and how they made me feel before I even did the cleanse. I reviewed the food families of the items in the diary, looking for patterns and trends in relation to how I felt. *Food families is a term used to group and categorize the foods we eat – fauna (the animals: bovine versus poultry versus fish, etc), flora (the plants: cruciferous versus citrus versus composite leaf (aka lettuces)), and fungi (mushrooms and yeasts).*

I determined which plants were in the same families and those that were in different families. I also made note of how often I found reactions related to recommended food combining rules; it made me see where I could improve. It was very enlightening to keep that food diary. Coupled with the review of my current blood work at the time, I identified the deficiencies in my diet choices. Adding that information to the diagnosis of arthritis I was able to map out a series of foods that were potential aggravations to my current health. Removing those offending families, I theorized which foods should make me feel better. This was my proving ground, the concept of food families and the elimination or addition of those family members to maintain my health. There is a good list of foods in Dr. Haas' book. However, it did not explain what it was in each food or its family that may be the trigger, the chemical composition which could be the irritant. I am the data geek, so in search of the data I went.

In the beginning, the lists that I used for my analysis were not entirely comprehensive enough so I went back to my scientific roots – and that meant research. Over the last three years have, I covered quite extensively details of the foods that I eat and what serves me best. I frequently scour the Internet for new studies and analyses on various foods that we eat. Along with this was a detailed analysis of their related food families.

I have consistently performed detoxification cleanses every quarter for the last three years. I try to make it follow the seasons, however with the kind of day job I have I'm lucky to stay within the season at all. Since my first cleanse in May 2009, I have tracked what I ate and been very strict to stay on a gluten, nightshade and soy free lifestyle. Those were the foods I identified to be my biggest culprits in causing my ill-health. After each cleanse I evaluated the exposure and consumption of the foods that I ate and tracked subsequent reactions. A few times a year, I found that I could consume dairy, just not on a consistent or rotational basis.

If you follow the concept that your body regenerates itself entirely every seven years; and your blood system every 90-120 days, and your skin every 21-30 days; then on a quarterly basis you should end up with a whole new 'clean' set of blood.. There are many things we consume repeatedly which will over time alter the way the cells regenerate. If you keep attacking the cells and triggering immune responses, the cells build up a wall of protection around them. The attack can be from infection, disease, immune deficiency, or actual toxin. The cells get bigger and because those triggers exist on a consistent basis. The new cells that get recreated have been 'programmed' (for lack of better terms) to be insulated.

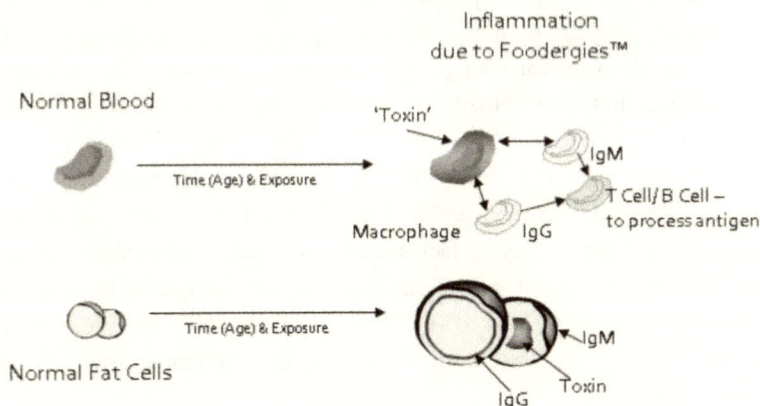

Inflammation
due to Foodergies™

Normal Blood

'Toxin'

Time (Age) & Exposure

IgM

Macrophage   IgG

T Cell/ B Cell –
to process antigen

Time (Age) & Exposure

Normal Fat Cells

IgM

IgG   Toxin

This programming can be reversed. The cells can learn to produce less and less insulation. Some of the 'toxins' or triggers come from Foodergies™ – our food foes. We don't always recognize the enemy until it makes its biggest impact to our health. I like to think of those 'toxins' that exist in our bodies' residing in our cells on a last-in, first-out philosophy. The most recent 'toxins' you consume or acquire should be the first ones that leave your body when performing a detoxification/cleanse. Years of buildup will take repeated cleanses to strip down and then come up to the surface for removal. Some 'toxins' come out easily since they are present in your bloodstream while others require breaking down of fat deposits for them to be released.

When I reflect back on all the things that I had tried early in my education, I realize how much I still did not know then but know now. One of those lessons I learned was trying a commercial diet system with packaged foods that were high in soy proteins. It was a failed experiment as I ended up having a soy allergy (IgE) with dermatitis based eczema. It took over six weeks of daily dosing of strong antihistamines to remove those hives and flakes from my body. Now of course, I know that I probably should've done heavy doses of histamine homeopathically, and a longer cleanse at the first sign of those eczema/hives. Back then I was following a traditional doctors and allergist's recommendations. There is nothing wrong with the approach or the solution provided by the allergist-it worked. But was it the most holistically supportive approach? Not entirely, as it was just a different way of approaching the problem – remove the symptom without finding the source of the allergy and properly eliminating and/or preventing hives.

So undergoing the cleanse, changing my diet and monitoring quarterly was quite a tall order for changing my lifestyle. I am not one to do things with less than full commitment; in fact it's usually all or nothing - so this was going to be a dedicated mastery of wills. I was tired of being in pain, ill health and stressed out from my IT project management job. As a professional project manager undertaking this level of project on a personal basis is not foreign to me. In fact, that was the way I was able to succeed with this new exercise of will. There's an old rule for quality management "say it, do it, prove it"- and to me, that meant plan your cleanse and diet, execute the plan, and document the effort. Quality management for my health meant:

- Finding the foods that supported my health and those that did not using the food families analysis – finding my Foodergies™.

- Pick the cleanse that will remove the most toxins each quarter (there are a few different types that work depending on your current state of health)

- Stick to your proper food list of food friends post cleanse and keep a food log, consistently

Seems pretty simple and straightforward - well for me it was. I would fall off the wagon during the experiment and would determine the kind of reaction of eating a "food foe" to determine if it was a food allergy or sensitivity. Once I actually expose myself to those non-serving foods, the trick was how to I counteract what I just did to myself. Sometime it is an herbal tea, green drink, homeopathic remedy, enzyme therapy and/or probiotic that will undo the effect of what I ate — it really depends on what the reactions are. Over the last three years I've gotten pretty good at catching any potential reactions before they get too bad. I have removed over 90% of my allergies — leaving just the anaphylactic few; even my prior debilitating pollen/ hay fever/ seasonal sinus and eye watering has been reduced to a minor seasonal mold/cold reaction in my eyes that lasts over the winter. I can count how many minimal cold or virus attempts and how many I have actually had on one hand in the last 3.5 years. Prior to cleaning up my Foodergies™, it was at least a dozen colds and 2-3 bouts of the flu a year. I am thankful to have my health back and have no intention of reverting back.

All this was done in the name of being able to support others as well as myself - going back to "Dr. Heal Thyself". Here I am a naturopath and health coach - who wants to be a good role model from the start — so I have to be able to "say it, do it, prove it" and educate others how to as well. So to summarize the suggested process:

  ⁊ Keep a food log for at least 2 weeks (30 days is optimal) tracking how you feel after meals along with any skin or respiratory reactions, pain or neuralgia, number of bowel movements and quality. The purpose of the bowel tracking is to determine the amount of Fiber and hydration in your current diet.

  I cannot stress how important tracking bowel movements is – it seems odd however the quality of your health depends on it. Dehydration causes self-toxification of our bodies — we do it to ourselves even if we supposedly eat really well. If you can't move it out of the colon efficiently, it festers and toxifies in you and that impedes your immunity. You can keep track of this information in a notebook or word processing file or an app on your iPhone/Android device; the operative phrase is **"keep a log"** – document, document, document.

    €&#x03; Review your food log for specific reactions and patterns with foods consumed and compare against the food families in this book.

    €&#x03; Organize your food consumed in a food map (see attached outline and sample).

    €&#x03; Based on the reactions flag those foods as supportive or derailing to your health goals. Supporting foods are kept and derailing ones are evaluated post cleanse.

    €&#x03; Perform a detoxification cleanse using vegan protein shakes, juice fasts, Dr. Cousens' Rainbow Diet, Dr. Haas Detox Diet or the Burrough's Master cleanse. There are other programs which use the foods we eat to detoxify and cleanse without supplementation or powders. Find one that works for you. For some of us, based on our current state of health at the time of the detox, a combination of styles may be the best way to go.

    €&#x03; Upon the completion of the cleanse, perform a dietary challenge/ elimination diet style exercise based on the 'Sensitive Seven" *(Sugar, Wheat, Dairy, Eggs, Corn, Soy, and Peanuts)* as per Dr. Haas. Your list may be the same as mentioned or modified based on your potential food foes (Foodergies™) documented in your food log.

It is not wise to immediately go back to the way you had been eating after a cleanse as the body needs to readjust to consuming foods that require more digestive processing. Easing back using broths, semi-soft foods and then migrating to more solid foods is suggested. Also, it is important to continue to avoid those foods you identified as not serving your best health for at least one week so that the body will not re-trigger an immune reaction. After that you may consume one serving of one of the potentially offending foods from your list and track for three days before attempting/trying another potentially offending food – for me it was a serving of bread, wait three days, then try dairy. Your body is the most receptive to potential sensitivities after a cleanse. As stated before, sensitivities can take up to three days to surface. This can continue for up to two weeks to fully analyze all the potential foods that may upset your health. This is a crucial point to focus on because you don't want to consume more than one as it could be the combination of the two or you may not be able to clearly discern which of the foods is causing the reaction. In the end, a consistent 4 day minimum rotation of the fringe Foodergies™ foods helps keep toxins and allergens consumed to a minimum.

There are many sources for performing an elimination/challenge diet. Please refer to the Supporting Documents and Links for those documents which detail how to perform an elimination/challenge diet.

80 Continue to document your food - the absence of the Foodergies™ (food foes) and increase of the food "friends" in your diet.

It is imperative to keep a positive mindset with respect to this whole exercise. When people function with limitations, it can be perceived as negative and restrictive, and the last thing you want to be feeling is that. I rather see it as an opportunity for growth and change. Small beneficial changes consistently beget longer lasting improvement.

My friends ask "Well, what *do* you eat?" I reply "I eat plenty of foods and there are those that just don't work for me anymore and plenty of others that do; let me share with you what does work versus what does not." There are specific foods that I do have to call out as verboten – like nuts, shellfish/Crustaceans, and gluten since I am celiac. There are some cheeses I can tolerate in small quantities though I choose not to consume voluntarily. The same can go for Soy or nightshades. The more I choose other foods versus these troublesome few the better off I am in the long run. But that's just me and this anecdotal description is used more for example so that you the reader may be able to craft your own analysis and determine what works best for you.

What state of health determines that cleanses can be beneficial?

Cleanses are important to help maintain digestive health for those with compromised immune systems and health. There is a segment of the population that says they are healthy enough so that cleanses seem like overkill or unnecessary. Our bodies have been in 'super-size' mode for over 20 years – the exposure of larger Coffees, larger sodas, larger fast food meals and the like. To consistently consume such enormous quantities is damaging to our health and cleanses are a good stop gap activity to halt the damage and start to reverse it. In the movie "Super-Size Me" it was medically proven that over consumption and especially fast food consumption is unhealthy. Also, in "Fat, Sick and Nearly Dead" the same message came across. How many people actually saw those films and thought, "Nah – I don't have those problems" and they actually do? In the end the most simplistic health improvement message paraphrased comes from Michael Pollan, from *In Defense of Food*, as 'eat not too much, mostly plants'. There is a lot to be said from that. Excess exists in our lives on many levels; stress, bad food options, caffeine, and portion sizes are some of the key culprits of excess. Well, if we have been conditioned to consume a lot, we have to deprogram ourselves and reset. The best course of action, for some, is a cleanse of some sort. Think of it like a Foodergies™ detox, like folks who are being detoxified from nicotine, narcotics, or alcohol addiction. Foods that hurt you or you have sensitivity to are essentially toxic. Want to start with a clean slate? Cleanse or Fast will do it.

I differentiate a cleanse versus a fast – a cleanse is a planned event of controlled consumption of foods with the end goal of resetting metabolism and digestion, e.g. Burroughs Master Cleanse. A fast is a deliberate event where abstinence and consumption of specific items is dictated to achieve spiritual or physical goals e.g. Daniel's Fast. I have seen "no-food, just water" fasts, fresh juices via juicer fasts, smoothies with just fruit fasts, fruit and vegetable smoothies, with and without protein powders and other amendments. There is a version for just about every personality, disposition of person and they may not work for everyone. Dr. Haas' The New Detox Diet has an excellent section on detoxification and fasting protocols.

Juice based fasts - I have people I know who are 100% dedicated to juicing and consumption with minimal manipulation of that juice afterwards. It works for them to reverse ill health and weight issues and is very inspiring. My scientific nature lauds the creativity of such an approach, however, juicing is a very modern concept. The first 'juicers" were geared around extracting nutrients from Wheat grass over 50 years ago. Blenders were used until someone figured out how to optimally extract nutrients through juice with minimal disruption of plant cellular structure. To amp up the completeness of the juices, proteins were extracted and concentrated and turned to powders, and then added back into the juices. Seems like a lot of work that a healthy set of teeth and jaw muscles could accomplish. It would help if we had enough digestive enzymes, sufficient stomach acid and proper gut flora to make this wonderful beverage work best for us.

Well, it seems we have hit the snag – obtaining those key desired results takes *time* and *patience*. In this lighting fast society, results not obtained quickly or in a 'reasonable' amount of time means the pattern of behavior is abandoned. So, if juicing is not working for you, or has been too time consuming, you stop. Same with any change in diet or cleanse. Consistency is key here; I cannot stress enough about preparation and commitment either. Success is based on those three elements and one can only work to the best supported path. Naturopaths, Health Coaches and Nutritionists are your best source of support and helping you "own" your health.

Most folks abandon during the first 72 hours of a cleanse or fast because of the 'healing crisis' symptoms or worsening of existing symptoms called Herxheimer reactions. These reactions are provoking an inflammatory response because the body is dumping the toxins in the bloodstream for elimination. Fasts cause a rapid break down of fat cells which drive the stored toxins from the fat stores into the bloodstream. Cleanses which target the digestive areas and liver can produce a slower increase of those toxins, making it longer before the reaction takes place. I can tell you this is absolutely normal and having done quite a few cleanses personally and from coaching others through them; I know how bad my toxins were that quarter by my reactions in that first 24-48 hours. I am usually on the other end of the phone or at their house, helping them through the monster headache that borders migraine levels, the skin itchiness, the muscle twitches, the body aches, the sniffles, and the feeling physically cold. Once they break the headache or 24-36 hours mark, everything starts to clear, like a fog lifting; they may get a burst of energy and want continue doing the cleanse longer. It is suggested to keep your first cleanse between 5-8 days.

There are those folks who are miserable the entire 5-8 days of the cleanse/fast and do not feel any difference. When questioned on the frequency of their bowel movements, most had very few movements. On occasion, there are folks who respond too well and have the 'melting' effect. The bowel responds with an irritated response and liquefies – diarrhea. It is not painful, just can catch you in an unpleasant surprise. I know in many cleanse and fast books they never mention that effect, and I have seen it happen. This means that the digestive system is not responding well and the 'melting' as well as the constipation can negatively impact the flora balance in the colon. These reactions can also be a reaction to the a food consumed that causes sensitivities (not previously identified) as part the cleanse/fast. This is where extra probiotics and neutral gentle fibers like inulin are added. Addition of this fiber at the outset and during the cleanse/fast will stop the melting. The body responds best when the toxins come out easily versus being backed up and irritating the colon or being flushed too quickly.

The optimal functioning gastrointestinal behavior as dictated by Dr. Bernard Jensen states one bowel movement should occur after every meal, which means three times a day we remove the waste from our bodies. Let's be honest how many people really do that? For some people, they are getting by with one every day to three days; others function 3 times a day and even some people move 5 to 6 times or more a day. Those digestive behaviors are all varying states of health and metabolism. A well known doctor stated during a broadcast that three times a **week** at minimum is considered normal and healthy. Really? Who is right? I strongly believe depending on what is consumed 'better out than in as efficiently as possible' means moving your bowels 2-3 times a day.

Over 80% of human immune system is managed by the gastrointestinal tract, specifically the small intestine. Due to diets of excess/overindulgence, the colon can become irritated, compromised and intestinal permeability may exist. That permeability impacts the quality of digestion as a whole, our immunity and the ability of our colons to do their job. The small intestine allow nutrients to enter the body, acts as a wall against parasite, microbial/ bacterial/ toxic waste and push that through to the large intestine and bowels to leave the body. If you add constipation to this permeability issue, it can become the source of one's inflammation and immunity challenges.

How does one reverse this condition, this internal inflammation? Identification, documentation, confirmation. It goes back to the "say it, do it, prove it" model. Identify the foods in their food families, document the reactions, eliminate them from your diet, reset your digestion, test and reevaluate the foods in confirmation. There are many theories many suppositions and many documented papers describing at length the best approaches to fixing oneself where immunity is concerned. Removal of pesticides, eating organic, maintaining healthy gut flora – these are all reactive actions when we are older and wiser. The education needs to take place with those adults before they have kids so that they can be better prepared for their child's future health.

Once your digestion is reset, performing tasks like what is mentioned is actually a more proactive approach to prevent repopulation of foreign materials, germs and dysbiosis in our digestive system. Repair of that permeability can take weeks to over a year depending on the age of the person, as well as duration and severity their symptoms. There are those to whom repair will not be as quick due to repeated re-exposure to those foodergies™ even in minute quantities. The colon takes approximately 2 years to regenerate in the body regeneration cycle, which is a lot longer than the skin or blood. Whatever we process through digestion will show up in our skin and blood faster than in our colon. Until the colon is healed, we will still be sending food toxins back into our blood and it may show up in our skin to be 'detoxified'. Foodergies™ – food allergies and sensitivities/intolerances – can be those toxins we struggle with identifying so that we can properly manage our diets and health.

Foodergies™ have patterns based on the food and its respective food family. The next sections go into each of the major groups of food families. There is an initial discussion of the family in a scientific way, the history of the foods where applicable and a complete list of commonly consumed family members. Additionally, there is a detailed analysis of the vitamins, minerals, amino acids and compounds found in those food members. There is also an explanation of why or why not an individual may want to consume these foods. These details were items I collected in my personal research which helped me understand what foods were my friends and which were potential foes. I wanted to know the **what** as much as the **why**, so that it made sense to me. During my analysis, it was important to know what impact the changes in food families did to my nutritional balance. If not eating specific foods led to potential deficiencies in my diet, I needed to find foods and their families to replace those missing nutrients as best as possible. For me, there were many food family to support what I gave up; just one or two could not be replaced completely by foods at all. I have listed my text and online references that were used so you could refer to them in your own research.

3 LET'S GET STARTED

So what is the deal with food families and how does it work?

We, the biologically unique, electro-chemical engines, need to know what food is the best fuel for each of us. That is why there are so many diets and lifestyle programs out in the market today. This book does not intend to focus on specific diet lifestyle programs, however it leverages and shares data from the *Eat Right for your Type* program by Dr. Peter D'Adamo, Nutrition Data reference section from Self.Com, Ayurvedic food combinations as well as a myriad of research sources available through PUBMED.com and GREENMEDINFO.com.

There is a lot to be said about our electro-chemical machines. Simply put, we function on a form of sugar which converted in our bodies into ATP. This fuel helps our bodies perform cellular respiration and send chemical connections which are carried through our bloodstream to instruct our bodies how to function on a second-by-second basis. Our blood types have evolved over time due to 'chemical' exposure to produce lectins which have been documented to react positively and negatively with the food we eat. Take a piece of apple, along with almond nut butter on a slice of whole grain bread – it sounds like a great snack, right? When that snack is processed by digestion, it ends up as that 'sugar', then fuel and chemical instructions. Each person will process the fuel and chemical instructions differently. This snack would harm some of my clientele, the apple may cause a reaction; the almond butter causing anaphylaxis; – a food allergy (IgE); where the whole grain bread is concerned - for me and some others, it is a food intolerant reaction that builds slowly, damaging the digestive system each time the whole grain (glutens) are attempted to be broken down. When evaluating the foods you eat and grouping them into food families, you can see the patterns of consumption and their potential antibody reactions in you. Classifying plants, animals and fungi into food families means they possess similar chemical structures i.e. proteins, alkaloids, sugars, toxins as part of their biological structure. I performed this research to support my own personal Foodergies™ issue. The more I shared about the lessons I had learned, it was evident this information was important to share. I was excited to share my results with my one client about his issues with apples, plums or peaches. It is similar to why I cannot have almonds (The answer is in Chapter 10 – Commonly Consumed Fruits and Vegetables). Sure makes me think I had better re-evaluate my eating apples too.

The epigenetic dilemma – why does eating 'hurt' our health?

How did we become a society of digestively challenged and immunity compromised individuals? True, not everyone suffers, however a large segment of the population has had challenges since the day they were born. What has happened to our 'machines' at birth that contributed to our immunity being compromised? There are soap boxes of opinions that can be leapt off from here and many books and papers that have been published on that subject. One of the earliest Naturopaths, Henry Lindlahr stated simply– "it is all about the soil." As a mother of two special needs boys, I heartily agree with that perspective. The "soil" being my body, the genes of the mother and father expressed – based on the diet of us both, and our current states of health at time of conception. Reflecting back on my health prior to both of my sons' births, the challenges I've had in my life, little did I know why or its source. I realize that parts of it became the "soil" that my sons would be born with.

Genetics is a funny thing, especially when you do a lot of postmortem digging through your data on a personal level. My genetic history has arthritis, allergies, high blood pressure, cardiovascular disease, addictions, and mental illness. My aunt suffered postpartum depression with her one and only pregnancy at age 38. Here I am reflecting on my own sons and seeing how my gene exposure is now expressed in them. I was fortunate not to have postpartum depression after the first pregnancy, though with my second, at the same age of 38, it reared its ugly head. In fact it was diagnosed late enough to cause significant impairment to my daily life. I've learned to question a normal blood test result because for me it was wrong for over two years. I did not want to be a guinea pig for modern medicine any longer. I vowed never to let this happen to anyone else so I went back to school and rededicated myself to learning and being ready to educate others.

That is how the die was cast that made my boys who they were at birth and their state of health. Their health was good while breastfeeding especially when I ate well. They had poor reaction to formula and specific food choices as they matured. Their state of health had certain 'factory settings' and I found that their diet could turn them on and off. I admit ruefully that their diet was especially poor before I 'woke up' to the food family relationships. My boys used to eat like every other standard American. Now there is a lot of negotiation on what they want and can and should eat as they are older. My elder son makes better choices every day, moving towards a 90 best/10 fun dietary perspective – he is about 70/30 and still moving up. The younger one still fights my suggestions which he perceives as limitations. He still does not see how the 90/10 works for him yet – it is a journey as he is 7 years younger than his elder brother and the same logic or Jedi mind tricks don't work on him. The elder is a high-functioning Asperger's autistic with ADD and slow processing. Initially I used muscle testing and followed up with IgG blood work to confirm what diet choices may work best for him. He was showing gluten and dairy intolerance, as well as a significant Candida issue. By adjusting my elder son's diet and removing those offending items, his health improved.

The changes in my elder son's diet, the acknowledgement of what eating certain foods does to him resonates more now than before. In fact, the outward symptoms of his conditions are becoming less observant to others. I would not say he is cured (yet, but every day closer) – however, I would like to say that with training, maturity and support along with diet – he is turning into a fine young man. I still have work to do with his brother. The elder one likes to help me "direct" his brother and I remind him it is about coaching and educating, **not** directing ☺.

My sons' diets have changed for their better health moving forward NOW before they are adults. I am cultivating their "soil" for their future. This lesson of epigenetics was learned out of love. Together we found feeding themselves better, fueling their engines for their best efficiency would be the support for wherever their brains/bodies want to take them. Retraining their diet and lifestyle now can "flip off" gene expression for the historical illness from both of their parents' gene pool and prevent the current ones from being "flipped on". This lesson goes back to you are what you eat, and how it impacts the future of your genes.

As adults. we can do the same thing – we can flip off the ones we inherited that can lead us to chronic and debilitating diseases. It may take longer depending on our current state of health and commitment level. There is no magic pill to make us better. There are medicines which can facilitate our bodies' abilities to heal as well as mask the symptoms for a while, but sometimes with side effects. There are scores of physicians and natural health practitioners who have proven that diet and lifestyle modifications "change" us – because we are reflecting the expression of the food choices we make and ultimately eat.

Over the last 4 years, the theory had to be "proven" to be the right choice for me and flexible for others. There has been a lot of observing and tracking the food families and how different it would be for every individual. I am a practitioner who uses muscle testing as an initial approach to facilitate the conversation of education on what can make the body weak. Muscle testing is non-invasive. I have used the muscle testing technique on myself and others for the last 3.5 years with great success. There are folks who question the results of this method with valid concern. The scientist in me likes to have lots of correlating data from many sources. I have suggested IgG/IgE/IgA blood work and DNA testing to be performed by their allergists, rheumatologists and/or primary care physicians to corroborate the muscle testing results. Once all those results together are reviewed, one can properly 'educate' on food families and Foodergies™, so that folks can improve their health.

How to use this book

Mother Nature provided food in the forms of animals and plants. The scientific classification of that set of animals and plants, otherwise known as fauna and flora, was documented by a man named Linnaeus. His work was shared with the scientific community in 1735. It is with this classification system that the foods we consume can be grouped into food families. Looking at the members of the food families you may find that it seems weird for some plants to have such differing members. An example is the cashew family has the following members: cashews, pistachios and mangoes - they sure doesn't seem like they could be related. Mother Nature has her reasons and the scientific community investigates and provides explanations as to why and reclassifies if necessary.

So, reflecting back on my skin issue - there was nothing wrong with the approach or the solution provided by the allergist for my case with my soy induced eczema. The goal of removing the eczema was achieved – or was it? Was it the most holistically supportive approach? Not entirely. The symptom and condition were treated. It took time for my skin to regenerate and body to remove the last of the toxins from the food I ate. If I had just gone back to eating soy after that incident, just not frequently, could I have had another skin episode? Yes – an IgE allergy was manifested so I would eventually have to repeat the same steps. I chose not to add anymore soy into my diet so I knew I was not fueling this food allergy or sensitivity flame. On occasion, I have the exposure to a bit too much soybean oil or soy lecithin and get a small bout of hives. I just change my diet and take a homeopathic at the onset and it is gone within 1-2 days, not months. I wish I knew more back then. I would have trusted my homeopathic instincts and just stayed the course to heal my eczema. It would have taken about the same amount of time, just the homeopathic remedy strength needed to be higher; that and I would have eaten more skin supportive foods too – leeks, pumpkin seeds, and flaxseeds.

In today's healthy food landscape - one day, broccoli is the savior, the next day it is kale or flaxseed. I predict parsley will be next. If you look up broccoli and kale in this book you will find they are part of the same major cruciferous vegetable family, though different branches. Parsley is not in this family at all and neither is flaxseed. This is some of the information that this book will educate and share with you: e.g., what makes broccoli, kale and parsley so important to our health and what it may do if your body happens to be sensitive to any of them. We *Homo sapiens* are inherently omnivores – we consume the flora (fruits, vegetables, tubers, herbs), fauna (animal products – beef, pork, fowl, game, fish, crustacean, bivalves), and fungi that exist on this earth. There are those foods which are now extensively genetically modified. Some of our foods have been bred over standard evolutionary patterns of plant and animal husbandry (also known as farming). We are fortunate that some foods are the same as they have been for hundreds of years.

If you want to know what could be your sensitivity or food issue – **document it**. Keeping a food diary is not that difficult, especially in the modern age. I have been keeping one for the last 3 years straight. I can tell you with utmost certainty what I ate, the reactions I had and most importantly, what I did to reverse them when they occurred. My food diary included what I ate and the quantities for the most part. I am not counting calories although I do keep a rough track. I am specifically counting categories of food families. I am observing dietary interactions similar to the food combining – proofs of the theory so to speak and how it worked with me and my engine. My most recent analysis surrounds food combining and food combination reactivity. Not a lot of attention has been paid to this topic and in each chapter, it is mentioned for each food family. Though I had been thorough with my documentation, there was not enough attention to food combination reactivity. It has become more evident with my reactions that foods combined properly can have a beneficial effect or not. When I get I hive or reaction which I cannot explain, it has pointed to some form of food combination that did not mesh well.

Those who desire this level of accuracy have to put in the time, honest disclosure of foods and reactions and repeat the challenge tests in controlled environments. It is work to do, to be consistent and be diligent. It is recommended for you to work closely with your health practitioner – Physician, Naturopath, Nutritionist or even a Health Coach to support you during this time to ensure the most accurate gathering of data. It pays off in the end with a clearer picture and direction to obtaining your best health possible.

> *Additionally, you can work with your practitioner to obtain an IgG blood test if you a looking for documented proof of sensitivity or intolerance. IgE (through skin prick or RAST) testing exclusively covers the standard "allergy" to a food or substance and is accessible to your Primary Care Physician or Allergist. There are quite a few organizations that have excellent track records of accuracy and informative nature. Please refer to the Sample Documents and References (Chapter 11) for a list of independent testing organizations.*

Part of the data collection should be a more detailed review of your blood type and family history of illnesses. When I donate blood and they check what I am, I come up as A positive. I am technically a mixed blood type – part A, part O but I show up as an A (my father was A and my mother was O). This is because O has no lectin expressions and it will take on the "mask" of what ever lectin is present. B blood types can be the same – part B/part O. As part of my Naturopathic studies on the many diets out there, I tried the A blood type diet by Peter D'Adamo. I was surprised how it did not work that well for me and at the time I did not know why. I had forgotten a piece of information my mother wrote in my baby book. She is a big fan of genetics and thought it was important to record that my father and she were different blood types. She had taught me a lot when I was 11 by using tropical fish as examples. The fish's body colors were more complex due to more gene combinations on a Mendel Plot than the preliminary assessment of blood types in humans. Once I located that information – I evaluated the O blood type diet too and found out I was a blend of the two. So, for me – the food families that keep me working smoothly are mixed between those that are A and O. I have the Celiac gene and nut/shellfish food allergies (IgE); I have early onset of arthritis documented in my family, lactose intolerance due to excessive antibiotics in my youth, as well as diabetes, dementia, heart disease and breast cancer. That is a lot of switches to turn off that got turned on due to my prior diet/lifestyle choices. Add that to a more unique combination of foods that suit me better, identifying this was extremely helpful to setting up a plan for my health.

A quick blood type history lesson: The first blood type documented by scientists was O – meat centric/hunter type. It was believed to be present starting 30,000 BC. Next on the scene was the introduction of an agrarian/cultivation type where farming and grain cultivation started – blood type A, occurring around 25,000 BC found in the European areas. The next blood type B was a more nomadic, flexible type originating in the Asia continent around 15,000 BC. The cultures intermingled more producing the rare AB around 2,500 BC in the Middle East and becoming more common about 1,000 years ago.

So for me, in examining the food families that are A and O supportive, you can see that my food choices and blood type coincide where those who are O have shown to be gluten/dairy sensitive, and meat eaters, while the A side of me could be totally content as a pescaterian (fish eating vegetarian). For folks who are B or AB your analysis of food families will have some similarities, differences and compromises. The omnivore formula works for me – free of gluten/dairy/nightshade/shellfish/soy, with limited beef/pork – more fish/fowl, and veggies/fruit families which are not nut related. Believe me, there is still plenty to eat and not be bored. In my household, with a professional barbeque chef, I find myself going through seasonal vegetarian/pescatarian to light omnivores every year. It sure does keep things interesting and there has been more overwhelming support especially in light of my positive health. Some of my cooking adventures have even surprised them as being really tasty and down right healthy and while being gluten, nut, soy and nightshade free and dairy reduced/free. However, that is another writing adventure to follow this one.

Essentially, there is no wrong way to approach this book. It can be used as a reference which shares knowledge about foods and their family members first and foremost. This information presented has been gathered from peer researched results, published references and anecdotal evidence with examples from my life and of some of my clients, with their permission, of course.

So what do our engines/bodies need?

The human engine requires the proper balance of proteins, carbohydrates and fats, adequate minerals, vitamins and amino acids that come from *real* food; the kind of food your grandmother or great-grandmother would recognize. At best we can hope for some reasonable minimally processed, commercially produced, non-GMO facsimile. Our bodies thrive on nutrient dense produce and animal proteins treated with care. I will be the first to say, I prefer to consume real food grown from my garden, or another farm that I support locally and not to eat packaged convenience foods. Reality of time, value of money, and our microwave society behavior prevents some of these choices from being made consistently or cost effectively. There are always options for food choices, and with education, better ones can be made. For example, not every one has time to grow their own foods in a garden, or treat the garden "organically" to ensure even more nutrient dense crops. You can participate in a Community Supported Agriculture group – food co-ops (www.localharvest.org/csa). This will help ensure that you eat locally and with the seasons, or just shop organic as possible in your own grocery store/health food store. Remember – your time spent for maintaining health pays dividends in longevity.

What does our current diet / lifestyle push us towards?

There are folks that I know who are sugar and caffeine addicts, and proudly say so. Both are really extremes of our systems – the overload of the primary fuel (glucose) that, when not utilized gets stored (as fat), regardless of how artificially amped up our metabolism is through the alkaloid toxin of caffeine. I confess that at a point in my younger life I was one – finishing a pot of coffee myself, having donuts and cookies and fueling my hectic consulting day job. Looking back on what I looked like - dark circles under my eyes, puffy complexion and skin tone, and slightly underweight – do I wonder why? I was not eating smartly, just fueling my engine poorly and it was still reasonably young. I was stealing my future health at the cost of my present extreme engine needs.

There are also the extreme foodies – those who eat to excess and are addicted to the joys of eating. I totally relate to that. I love to eat good food, prepared with care, love and positive energy – I just don't eat out or consume those rich foods that much anymore, or even at one sitting. I would consider myself a reformed extreme foodie. I go out to eat though (not as frequently) watching for Foodergies™ with care along with the portion size. Having been at extremes in my food consumption - a strict vegetarian and ultimate carnivore, and places in between numerous times over my lifetime – I have found a reasonable plan with balance to fuel my body's needs. I am still fine tuning; the engine is older now and has different needs due to my careless treatment in my younger and middle years.

There are those who are so adrenal fatigued and depleted that they live on 5-Hour Energy drink. I have seen an enormous number of those bottles laid out on top of folks' cubicles, stacked 4 rows high (with pride mind you), all around the four sides – this image saddens me immensely. These people cannot function anymore without it; another addiction of excess. It may be only 5 calories and has missing vitamins, so how can it be addicting? Sure it can, because the body is so stressed out, and hormonally depleted. This liquid temporary fix is nothing more than a band-aid on a mortal wound. Stress in our human engine, in the form of free-radical and oxidative stress at the cellular level, causes overload, short circuiting and eventual burnout. Craving this kind of fix of energy on a consistent basis is like a large warning flag on the racetrack – a race car running in the red zone. At some point, no amount of quick shots of liquid booster cables will start that engine up, then where to turn? Back to what was there for us all along – real food, with nutrients, versus chemically derived ones.

We also have food cravings – lots of different kinds of them. My reasoning is thus – excess consumption of a specific food/toxin leads us down two pathways:

1) To deficiencies of key components of our health
2) An addiction to the chemical/toxin that it becomes a part of the vicious cycle of ill health.

One way or another in our diets, excess is the enabler and education with willpower is the disabler. Cravings can be alarms too – when we are deficient in something, our body may send us message to eat a food we normally would not to obtain the missing elements. A dear friend of mine normally would not have a piece of salmon for any reason. She did not know if she is allergic, or sensitive, but she does not like how she feels after eating it (sluggish). One day at lunch with her husband, the vision of the grilled salmon platter could not be avoided – like foot-high neon lights screaming '"Eat Me". To her husband's surprise and hers, she ate it with no ill effects – in fact she felt immensely better than before lunch. This was a case of the body letting us know what it wanted and needed desperately and happily reciprocated when consumed.

This is another one of those soap-box preaching detours I could go on, and I will abstain from the rant. My experience is that the Standard American Diet fails us in so many ways. I believe we need to eat the best clean foods available that serve our bodies, get physical exercise – not just mental, relax and reduce the free-radicals/toxins we get exposed to – and then we are on the way towards improving your health. Even doing half of this is better than nothing but the key to success is **consistency**. So start small, crowd out the foodergies™ and things that do not help your health. Then fill it with those foods and behaviors that do, and eventually there is nothing too bad left to deal with. I will be the first to say it is ok to fall off the wagon, once in a while, I know what it takes to get back on. I recently completed my Health Coaching Certification with the Institute of Integrative Nutrition in NYC and one of their mantras is the 90/10 rule: paraphrased as 90% of the time stick to it – 10% of the time, let yourself off the leash and enjoy in moderation. For me – falling off the wagon and eating gluten, nuts or nightshades hurts too much, and can injure, if not kill me. Too much soy on a consistent basis gives me hives and dairy gives me digestive issues. However one day of it (not both on the same day) spaced out here and there – is all OK. I can remediate with better food days, homeopathic remedies, probiotics and enzymes in between until my next cleanse. This is how I maintain my health. Now it is your turn to learn and see what you need for yourself.

Food Families – Short List

If you find you have sensitivities with a member of a certain food family, it would be considered wise to eliminate all others, in that family or at least cut back on them. The food family members possess similar chemical structures (i.e. proteins, alkaloids, sugars, and toxins) though their "packaging" is similar or different. Even mild consumption can be found to cause reactions, even in the smallest of quantities. It is the little bit from lots of the same family which end up being the source of the biggest irritation. For example – there is a difference in my reactions even between species of apples, whether they are conventionally or organic grown.

This is a recommendation not a rule as not everyone has the same allergy, sensitivity or intolerance. As biochemical individuals, unique to our genes, it is best during dietary elimination and testing/evaluation to make note of these families and document any interrelationships. The number of plants and animals we consume from all over this world can be pretty overwhelming. This list is the most complete reflecting current and commonly consumed foods as per all the research online and in books. Plants get reclassified based on analyses and there may be updates after the publication of this book. Families and specific members of a family that are marked with an ^ are available on the web at http://www.keileswellnesscare.com/foodfamilysummary.html. This web page will describe the benefits and drawbacks of consuming those other members of those food families.

Fauna – Animals and by-products

Dairy: Cow's milk and all foods derived from cow's milk, such as cheeses, yogurt^, kefir and cottage cheese^. Note: Butter is an exception as it tends to be less reactive, relatively low in milk proteins, and mostly fat. Other dairy products can be derived from Bovidae animals – yak milk^, goat milk^, and sheep milk^. Eggs are traditionally inferred as hen's eggs, though any member of Galliformes egg could be used.

Animal Meats

Family Bovidae – Cattle: Beef, Veal^, Bison^, Buffalo^, Yak^, Water Buffalo^, Goat, Lamb, Mutton^

Family Cervidae – Deer (Venison), Elk^, Moose^, Caribou^, Reindeer^

Family Leporidae^ – Rabbit, Hare

Family Suidae – Pig (Pork, Ham, Bacon, Sausage^, Lard^)

Poultry – Order Galliformes
  – Family Anatidae – Duck: Duck and Goose^
  – Family Columbidae^ – Pigeon: Pigeon, Squab and Dove
  – Family Odontophoridae^: New World Quail
  – Subfamily Family Phasianinae - Pheasant: Chicken, Cornish Hen^, Pheasant^, and Partridge^
  – Family Scolopacidae^ – Snipe: Snipe and Woodcock
  – Subfamily Family Tetraoninae – Grouse: Grouse^, Turkey, Guinea Fowl^
  – Order Struthioiniformes^ - Ostrich

Other Animals^

Family Ursidae: Bear

Family Macropodidae: Kangaroo

Crocodiles^

Family Alligatoridae: Alligator
Family Crocodylidae: Crocodile

Reptiles^

Order Chelonii: Turtle, Terrapin

Family Viperidae: Rattlesnake

Amphibian^

Order Anura: Frog

Seafood and Fish

Phylum Actinopterygii – Bony Fishes:
- Flounder: Flounder^, Halibut^, Sole, Turbot^, Dab^, Plaica^ (flatfish)
- Scombridae
  - o Mackerel: Mackerel, Albacore^, Mahi Mahi^, Yellowtail^, Tuna
  - o Bonito^
- Butterfish^, Hoverfish^, Swordfish^
- Jack^: Pompano^, Yellow Jack^
- Croaker^: Sea Trout, Weakfish, Silver Perch, Croaker
- Cod: Cod (Scrod), Haddock^, Pollack^, Hake^, Whiting^
- Herring: Sardine, Sea Herring^, Shad (roe)^
- Salmon: Trout^, Salmon
- Sea Bass: Grouper^, Sea Bass (White), Rockfish^
- Bass^: Bass, Yellow Perch, Snapper
- Minnow^: Carp, Chub
- Perch^: Sauger, Walleye Pike
- Sunfish^: Black Bass, Sunfish, Crappie
- Pike: Pike^, Pickerel^, Muskellunge^, Whitefish
- Catfish: Basa^, Bullhead^, Swai^, Lake Catfish
- Ocean Catfish^
- Mullet^: Mullet, Barracuda
- Sturgeon^
- Smelt^

- Anchovy^
- Sailfish^: Marlin, Sailfish
- Tilefish^
- Porgy^: Porgy, Red Snapper
- Eel^
- Tilapia^

Phylum Crustacea – Crustacean: Crab, Shrimp, Lobster, Crayfish^, and Prawns^

Phylum Chordata^ – Class Chondrichthyes: Cartilaginous Fish – Sharks, Rays, Skates, and Dogfish

Phylum Mollusca – Mollusks

- Gastropods: Abalone^, Conch^, Snails
- Cephalopods: Squid, Cuttlefish^, Octopus^
- Pelecycpods: Clam, Oyster, Scallop, Mussel, Cockles^, Winkles^

Flora - Plants
Grasses & Grains

Family Poaceae (True Grasses):
- Grain – Wheat^, Wheat Grass^, Rye^, Spelt^, Oats^, Triticale^, Kamut^, Durum, Bulgur^ and Barley
- Corn – Corn, Maize^, Blue Corn^, Popcorn^, Grits^
- Rice – White Rice^, Brown Rice, Basmati^, Jasmine^
- Sugars – Cane Sugar and Sorghum^
- Lemongrass^ – Lemongrass, Citronella
- Teff
- Millet
- Bamboo^
- Wild Rice

Family Amaranthaceae – Goosefoot/Spinach:
- Spinach
- Beet, Sugar Beet^, Chard

- Amaranth, Lamb's Quarter^
- Quinoa

Family Polygonaceae – Buckwheat:
- Buckwheat
- Rhubarb
- Sorrel

Legumes

Family Fabaceae / Leguminosae – Legumes (Bean and Pea):
- Soybean
- Haricot Beans (Phaseolus) – Green Bean (Snap Bean), Lima Bean, Butter Bean, Common Bean, Black Bean, Kidney Bean, Red Bean, White Bean (Cannellini or Navy Bean), Cranberry Bean, Pinto Bean, Spotted Bean^, Runner Bean^
- Peas – Snow Pea, Sugar Snap Pea, Common Pea^ (Mangetout Peas – eaten whole with pod before maturity)
- Alfalfa^
- Acacia^, Senna^
- Carob
- Chickpeas
- Peanut
- Licorice^
- Adzuki (Azuki) Bean, Black Eyed Pea^, Mung Bean^
- Broad Bean^, Fava Bean^, Lentil
- Fenugreek^
- Red Clover^
- Jicama
- Tamarind^
- Lupin^
- Mesquite^
- Tragacanth^
- Tonka Bean^

Fruits, Vegetables, Nuts, Seeds and Spices

Family Actinidiacea: Kiwi

Family Adoxaceae^: Honeysuckle - Elderberry (also known as Sambucus)

Family Algae^: Seaweed (Kelp), Kombu, Dulse, Carageenan, Agar

Family Amaryllidaceae: Onion, Garlic, Chive^, Green onions^/Scallion^, Leek, Ramp^, Shallot^

Family Anacardiaceae – Cashew:
   – Cashew
   – Pistachio
   – Mango
   – Poison Oak^, Poison Ivy^, Poison Sumac^

Family Annonaceae^: Soursop (guanabana), Sweetsop, Cherimoya, Atemoya, and Custard Apple

Family Aquifoliaceae^: Holly – Yerba Mate

Family Araceae^ – Taro:
   – Konjac
   – Taro, Poi

Family Arecaceae – Palm:
   – Cabbage Palm^, Acai^
   – Sago^
   – Dates
   – Palm oil^, Coconut

Family Asparagaceae – Asparagus:
   – Asparagus
   – Agave^, Yucca^

Family Betulaceae – Birch:
   – Filberts, Hazelnuts
   – Wintergreen^

Family Brassicaceae – Cruciferous Greens or Mustard:
- Arugula
- Watercress^
- Capers^
- Brassica Species
  o Oleracea groups
    ▪ Cauliflower, Broccoflower^
    ▪ Kale, Collard greens^
    ▪ Cabbage
    ▪ Brussels sprouts^, Savoy cabbage^, Chinese Kale (wild cabbage)^
    ▪ Broccoli
    ▪ Kohlrabi^
    ▪ Chinese Broccoli^
  o Turnip, Broccoli Rabe^, Chinese Cabbage/Napa^, Mizuna^, Rapini^
  o Rapeseed oil (canola)^
  o Rutabaga (also known as Yellow turnip^)
  o Mustard Greens^
- Horseradish^
- Wasabi^
- Radish, Daikon^
- Virginia Pepperweed^, Maca Root, Garden Cress^

Family Bromeliaceae: Pineapple

Family Cactaceae^ – Prickly pear cactus, Dragon fruit

Family Cannabaceae – Hemp Seed, Hops^

Family Capparaceae^ – Caper Berry

Family Caricaceae – Pawpaw: Papaya; Papain

Family Clusiaceae^ – Mangosteen, Mammee Apple

Family Convolvulaceae: Morning Glory – Sweet Potato

Family Compositae – Daisy Composite flower:
- Lettuce (Romaine, Red leaf, Green Leaf, Butter/Bib), Celtuse^
- Chicory, Endive, Escarole, Radicchio
- Globe Artichoke
- Sunflower, Jerusalem Artichoke^
- Yacon^
- Safflower^
- Chamomile^
- Dandelion
- Tarragon^, Mugwort^, Sagebrush^ (Absinthe), wormwood^ (Absinthe)/Vermouth^
- Arnica^
- Cornflower^
- Coneflower^ (Echinacea)
- Black Salsify^
- Yarrow^
- Burdock root^
- Goldenrod^
- Tansy^
- Ragweed^
- Milk Thistle^

Family Cucurbitaceae – Gourd:
- Crookneck Squash, Butternut Squash, Acorn Squash, Spaghetti Squash (Winter Squashes), Pumpkin, Summer Squash, Zucchini (Courgette)^
- Melons
  o Muskmelon^
  o Watermelon, Citron Melon^
  o Cantaloupe, Persian Melon^
  o Casaba Melon^, Honeydew, Crenshaw^
  o Bitter Melon^
  o Cucumber
- Winter Melon (Chinese Watermelon)^
- Chayote/Mirliton^

Family Cyperaceae^ – Water chestnut

Family Dioscoreaceae – Yam

Family Ebenaceae^ – Persimmon

Family Ericaceae – Heath/Bilberry:
- Blueberry, Cranberry, Cowberry^, and Huckleberry^
- Wintergreen^

Family Euphorbiaceae^ – Spurge:
- Cassava / Manioc / Yuca, Tapioca
- Castor Bean

Family Fagaceae – Beech/Chestnut: Chestnuts, Beechnut^ and Oak Acorns^, Chinquapin^

Family Grossulariaceae^: Saxifrage – Blackcurrant, Redcurrant, Whitecurrant, and Gooseberry

Family Iridaceae - Iris^: Saffron, Orris root

Family Juglandaceae - Walnut: Butternut^, Hickory nut^, Black Walnut, English Walnut, Pecan

Family Lamiaceae^ (or Labiatae) – Mint:
- Balm
- Basil
- Catnip
- Hoarhound
- Japanese Artichoke
- Lavender
- Marjoram, Oregano
- Mint, Peppermint, Spearmint
- Rosemary

- Sage, Chia
- Savory
- Thyme

Family Lauraceae – Laurel:
- Avocado
- Bay leaf^
- Cinnamon
- Sassafras (Filé Powder)^

Family Lecythidaceae: Brazil nut

Family Liliaceae^: Sarsaparilla

Family Linaceae: Flaxseed (Linseed)

Family Lythraceae: Pomegranate

Family Malpighiaceae^: Acerola

Family Malvaceae – Cola Nut: Chocolate^, Cacao^, Cocoa, Hibiscus^, Okra, Durian^, Cola nut^, Cotton^, Sterculia^, Gum Karaya^

Family Marantaceae^: Arrowroot

Family Moraceae – Mulberry: Mulberry, Fig, Jackfruit^, Bread fruit^

Family Musaceae – Banana: Banana and Plantain

Family Myrtaceae^: Myrtle – Allspice, Clove, Guava, Myrtle, Gum Acacia, Pimento and Pomarosa

Family Oleaceae – Olive: Green and Black olive, Jasmine^

Family Orchidaceae^ - Orchid: Vanilla

Family Oxalidaceae^: Carambola/ Star Fruit

Family Papaveraceae^: Poppy seed

Family Passifloraceae^: Passion Fruit

Family Pedaliaceae: Sesame seed

Family Pinacea: Juniper^, Pine nuts/Pignoli

Family Piperaceae^ – Peppercorn, Black and White Pepper

Family Portulacaceae^: Purslane

Family Proteaceae – Macadamia Nut

Family Rosaceae – Rose family: Blackberry, Boysenberry^, Dewberry^, Loganberry^, Raspberry, Youngberry^, and Rosehip^, Strawberries (their own subfamily within Rose family)

    Amygdaloideae sub family –
    – Genus Prunoideae - Plum: Plum, Prune^, Cherry, Almond, Nectarine^, Apricot, Pluot^, Sloe^ and Peach, Aronia^
    – Genus Maloideae - Apple: Apple, Pear, and Quince^, Medlar^, Loquiat^; Crabapple^, Apple Cider Vinegar^

Family Rubiaceae – Madder: Coffee, Quinine^, Ipecuahana^, Noni^

Family Rutaceae – Citrus: Grapefruit, Lemon, Lime, Orange, Tangerine, Tangelo^, Citron^, Ugli^, Clementine^, Pomelo^, and Kumquat^

Family Sapindaceae^ – Soapberry: Maple Sugar, Maple Syrup, Lychee and Rambutan

Family Solanaceae – Potato (Nightshades): Potato, Belladonna (Homeopathic Remedy of Deadly Nightshade plant)^, Tomato, Eggplant (Aubergine), Peppers (bell, red, green, chile, cayenne), Tomatillo, Paprika^, Goji Berry^, Cape gooseberry^ and Tobacco^

Family Theaceae - Tea^: Tea, Camilia

Family Umbelliferae – Carrot: Parsley, Parsnip, Carrot, Celery, Celeriac, Caraway^, Anise^, Dill^, Fennel^, Aniseed^, Cumin^, Coriander^, and Cilantro^

Family Vitaceae – Grape: Grape, Muscatels^, Muscadine^, Sultanas^, Currants, Raisin; Champagne^, Wines^, Brandy^, Sherry^, Cream of Tartar^ and Buckthorn tea^

Family Xanthorrhoeaceae^ – Aloe vera

Family Zingiberaceae: – Cardamom^, Galangal^, Ginger, and Turmeric^

Fungi

Fungi kingdom: Mushrooms, Puffballs^, Truffles^, Morels^, Chanterelles^, Quorn^, Mycoprotein^, Brewer's Yeast and Baker's Yeast

Preface to the Reference chapters: In each of the subsequent sections, food families are grouped then discussed at the 'family' level detail. If a food family states **"High in Vitamins"** *or* **"High in Minerals"** *as* **None**, *it does not mean there are no vitamins or mineral in that food family. It means that there is no largely significant (over 50% of RDA) value present. The same statement can be made for Key Chemical components in specific food families Also, when listing the High in Vitamins or Minerals, they may not be in alphabetical order; they may be in listed in higher quantity to lower quantity.*

If there are any questions about what is posted, feel free to send an email to foodergies@gmail.com *for clarification of information provided in the book. There is also a Foodergies™! Online forum:* **foodergies.forumcommunity.net** *for in-depth analyses on these families, desired improvements and additions to the book.*

4 GRASSES & GRAINS

The Family **Poaceae** (True Grasses) is the home of the plants we know as "whole grains." This food family is under investigation in over 200 major analyses, papers and articles as one of the key sources of the onset of most major illnesses. Yes, as the public we are led to believe that those whole grains are healthy for us. Whole grains are really the seeds of grasses or other plants that are "grain" like. It is a conundrum at best – to eat or not to eat and why. There are pro's and con's of every food family. One man's cure is another man's toxin – and for those who are Celiac or have other inflammatory conditions – this may be your issue. Let's start with the basics of botany and biology for this family then provide the pro's and cons of consuming plants from this family.

I am certified Gluten Free Practitioner and I have one of the two primary celiac genes (HLA-DQ8). I used to suffer from digestive issues, many food and pollen allergies and had weight issues until I stopped eating the primary group* of the family of Grass/Grain plants – Poaceae. For 2.5 of the last 3.5 years, I was diligent to keep all of it out of my diet, even in teas. My favorite coffee replacement tea, Roastaroma, uses roasted barley and I even stopped consuming that, just to keep all those issues at bay. I still consumed corn and rice on a limited basis and reduced my sugars and consumed mostly psuedocereals. It became evident as I started having minor episodes six months ago that corn was the next to go; soon it may be rice, quinoa or buckwheat. I do know what it means to be 'grass free' however instinctually, it does not feel that it may be right for me.

> *I understand how damaging those plants can be for some, if not most of us, even with the myriad of studies out there and their less than favorable results. As a scientist, I reserve the right of bioindividuality assessment to drive how "gluten free" a client could be, even for myself. When in doubt, I fully support GO WITHOUT GRASSES/GRAINS. Where there is IgG and genetic tests showing a specific grass/grain is permitted, even with Gluten Sensitivity/Intolerance or Celiac documented results, I would still that keep that food on a minimum 4 day rotation basis of a client's dietary plan. If the symptoms or illness have not improved with the removal of everything else but those very few, then 100% gluten free will be recommended.*

Grass -- *Family Poaceae* (True Grasses): There are many plants we call grains which are really seeds from grasses. These are consumed in various forms in our world – from primary consumption as flour, turned into breads to fillers/extenders in our medicines and foods.

The subgroups within this family are:

- ***Grain – Wheat, Wheat Grass, Rye, Spelt, Oats, Triticale, Kamut, Durum, Bulgur and Barley**. These are the primary group of grasses that called "grains." Genetic enhancement and manipulation to reduce growing time make it capable of being grown in different climates outside of the "course of nature." That behavior has made this group one of the most altered from native state plants which we consume today. Second and third are Soybeans and Corn.

- **Corn – Corn, Maize, Blue Corn, Popcorn, Grits**. Corn is a vegetable and called "sweet corn" but is still part of the grass family. Genetic manipulation for resisting disease and extended growing or hardiness has been more prevalent in the last 50 years.

- **Rice – White Rice, Brown Rice, Basmati, Jasmine**. Rice is technically the seed of the grass. Genetically, there are two sources of rice – Asian and African. Various native genetic cultivars exist before the advent of genetic modification. There are documented cases of modified gene expression to fill in nutritional gaps, however it could be perceived as true manipulation versus extended evolution.

- **Sugars – Cane Sugar and Sorghum.** These plants stalks are what are used to extract the sucrose for consumption. Due to large demand for sugars, sugar beets (another grass family member) are being used.

- **Lemongrass - Lemongrass, Citronella.** These plants are used for their oils not their seeds.

- **Teff** – A native South African grass seed used similarly as Bulgur

- **Millet** – A European grass seed used similarly to Teff and Bulgur

- **Bamboo** – These plants are consumed for their shoots from the stalks.

- **Wild Rice** – These plants are not remotely related to their cousins' African or Asian Rice. These grasses are North American native and used similarly as regular rice and are more fiber/nutrient rich.

High in Vitamins – Thiamine, Niacin, B6, E (in Wheat Germ).

High in Minerals – Copper, Magnesium, Manganese*, Phosphorus, Selenium and Zinc.

Amino Acids Completeness – Primary group of Grasses "whole grains" have an incomplete amino acid profile; other additional proteins need to be consumed to support necessary amino acid requirements in your diet.

Consumption Profile	Wheat, Durum raw 1 cup (192 g)	Corn, Sweet, Yellow raw (100 g)	Rice, Brown raw 1 cup (185 g)
Protein	26.2 g	3.2 g	14.7 g
Fat	4.7 g	1.2 g	5.4 g
Carbohydrates	147.0 g	19.0 g	143.0 g
Fiber	0.0	2.7 g	6.5 g

Consumption Profile	Cane Sugar brown (100 g)	Teff uncooked 1 cup (193 g)	Millet uncooked 1 cup (200 g)
Protein	0.1 g	25.7 g	22.0 g
Fat	0.0 g	4.6 g	8.4 g
Carbohydrates	98.1 g	141.0 g	146.0 g
Fiber	0.0 g	15.4 g	17.0 g

Consumption Profile	Barley, pearled raw (100 g)	Wild Rice raw 1 cup (160 g)
Protein	9.9 g	23.6 g
Fat	1.2 g	1.7 g
Carbohydrates	77.7 g	120.0 g
Fiber	15.6 g	9.9 g

Key Chemical components – Members of the Grass family possess a special structure called prolamine. This is part of the protein of the grass seed, also known as "grain", which is then ground to make our flours. It is found in the bran component of each plant. This prolamine structure is named differently for each member of the Grass family. Below is a chart of some of the key Grass family members, the name of the prolamine and the percent of the protein that prolamine takes up:

Grain/Grass	Prolamine	% Total Protein
Wheat	*Gliadin*	*69*
Rye	Secalinin	30-50
Oats	Avenin	16
Barley	Hordein	46-52
Millet	Panicin	40
Corn	Zien	55
Rice	Orzenin	5
Sorghum	Kafirn	52
Teff	Penniseiten	11

Note: in the previous chart, those that are shaded have the highest concentrations of prolamine. The largest by far is in Wheat – Gliadin. Essentially, the prolamine part of the "gluten" of the grass, which is the chemical trigger for "gluten sensitivity" in the Grass family. Gluten is actually a two part protein structure – prolamines and glutelins. Prolamines are alcohol soluble and the glutelins are broken down with weak acids or base solvents. You have heard that oats and rice are "gluten" free. Well, not exactly – their ratio of "glue" to protein is the least of the list above and that does not make it "free." Free of Gliadin, this is wheat specific – absolutely true, however free of prolamines – **not true**.

Additionally, when the proteins break down they release a natural opiate called gliamorphin which has been known to impact mental health as well. Our bodies utilize a chemical **Dipeptidyl peptidase-4** (DPPIV) to neutralize the opiate and it is found in the villi of the small intestine. However if our colons are compromised or there is an inherent sensitivity/intolerance, our bodies may not have enough DPPIV and the opiate can leak through into the bloodstream resulting in neurological imbalances. There are enzymatic supplements that contain DPPIV especially for those gluten triggered (and dairy triggered – casomorphin) impacted folks to help with the assimilation and digestive processing.

I believe this is the biggest confusion behind the gluten free lifestyle and maintenance of one's health. Wheat and its family members are EVERYWHERE and in the majority of things we eat. For those who have issues with it, cross contamination through various sources is a real threat to maintaining one's health – from starches used in medicines and drugs as binders, to fillers in foods, even in shampoos and conditioners. Remember the skin is the largest detoxification organ in our body – just as easily as toxins come out, they can go in – through the skin and enter the bloodstream, and then the immune response kicks in. The food toxin is the result of breaking down the protein (prolamine/gluten) and whether the body can process/assimilate its nutrients. It is a chicken-egg conundrum – does the person have inflammatory issues because of this inability to break it down genetically (or due to other gut permeability) or is the over consumption of genetically modified grasses or other proteins hyper stimulated the immune response that it making grasses "the enemy" as well as other foods, hence compromising the efficiency of the colon?

Education is key. Know about the things you consume – especially the packaged, processed stuff. I have been working to reduce the amount of packaged and processed foods in my household and it is not an easy task. The fewer ingredients and that are identifiable and are known the better. For example – STARCH is an added product to a lot of packaged/processed goods. Starch could from one of many sources: corn, wheat, rice, potato or tapioca. Do not assume if starch is listed with a rice based product, that it is a rice starch. On the packed "gluten-free" products, they are required to document the source of the starch and the packaging environment. Be careful of the "gluten free ingredients" but not a "gluten free facility" – that is one area that needs to be improved on, as cross contamination is no joke.

Thank you to the education I have received from Dr. Peter Osborne in my Gluten Free Practitioner certification and the data mining by Sayer Ji at GreenMedInfo for keeping me apprised of all the new studies and research on this topic.

Reasons to consume: The primary health benefits of grasses are the fiber component of the plant. A high fiber, low cholesterol diet with whole grains is supposed to help with cardiovascular and digestive health. Grasses also have natural Omega-3 and 6 essential fatty acids (EFA) as well as Ferulic Acid (an antioxidant which helps reduce inflammation), plant sterol/stanol esters.

Specific (purple/black/red) colored species of rice contain anthocyanins and tocols which possess antioxidant properties. These anthocyanins have shown retardation of plaque in the arteries when compared to other forms of rice.

Wheat bran is one of the best forms of constipation reliever. It is beneficial to the colon by bulking up the stool, diffusing toxins and keeping them away from the lining to potentially pass back into the bloodstream.

Reasons not to consume: Grass glutens may be the true source of your body's irritation that you consume multiple times a day. For some, it is the cause of pain and neurological instability; others it is hives and digestive impairment; or it is all of the above. Grasses are also high on the glycemic index as well, impacting the ability to metabolize sugars in our bodies efficiently.

If you have been genetically identified with the HLA-DQ2 or HLA-DQ8 genes, you have the capability of acquiring Celiac disease. There are also secondary genes which are the identifiers for intolerance/sensitivities (Beta from of the Alpha DQ2/DQ8). Once you have been identified, it is best to keep all grasses out of your diet. If desired, you may consider IgG immunity testing for which grass prolamines, if any, you can consume due to your genetic/environmental background. Detailed IgG tests are not your traditional "allergy" tests because they test a mature immune response which is more of an intolerance or sensitivity. An overall IgG response summary test is available through standard serum draws at your practitioner's office or draw center. Information about detailed IgG and Genetic Testing organizations is found in Chapter 11 of this book.

Phytic acid is found in the bran and the germ of grass seeds, especially brown rice. It does the body a service to bind with metals and chelate the bloodstream, however it can do it too well, leaching beneficial minerals and enzymes. This reduces our ability to break down protein and sugars and enabling the digestion in the small intestine. For those already digestively compromised folk, consuming something that has phytic acid as part of something 'healthy' is actually compromising your health further.

Additionally, key members of this food family (rice, corn, and wheat) have been genetically modified at length to produce plants in order to enable rapid maturity, pest/microbial management, and modify gene expression to produce non-original chemical compounds (e.g. rice that has been modified to express proteins found in breast milk or produce Vitamin A). Genetic modification to these lengths produce plants which can be seen as foreign to our bodies, further compromising our immune systems during the digestive process.

PSEUDO-GRAINS

Other "Grass" family members produce seeds which are consumed like grains, and the consumption of them is considered "gluten free" by the nutritional community. **Remember – all grasses have "glutens" just how much is in question and how your body reacts to them.** Certain genetic backgrounds evolved around these grains instead of wheat, corn or rice; how those proteins interact in our bodies is the same.

Buckwheat -- *Family Polygonaceae*: Plants in this family are buckwheat, rhubarb, and sorrel. Buckwheat is the plant which produces the grain like seeds also known as Kasha. This grain is commonly used in China, Japan and Russia.

High in Vitamins – Folate, Niacin.

High in Minerals – Copper, Magnesium, Manganese*, Phosphorus and Zinc.

Amino Acids Completeness – Buckwheat is just a bit short of the complete amino acid profile; a small amount of other proteins need to be consumed to support necessary amino acid requirements in your diet.

Consumption Profile	Buckwheat 1-cup (170g)
Protein	25.5 g
Fat	5.8 g
Carbohydrates	122.0 g
Fiber	17.0g

Key Chemical components – Has Omega-3 and 6 Essential Fatty acids (low Omega-3/6 Ratio); phenolic/antioxidant compounds of Rutin (a break down product of Quercetin) and tannins; also has key phytosterols – Beta-sitosterol, Campesterol, Stigmasterol, which reduces cancer risk, prostate inflammation and LDL cholesterol levels.

Reasons to consume: Rutin is a phytochemical that strengthens capillary walls; the high protein component of buckwheat has been shown to reduce plasma cholesterol, body fat, and cholesterol gallstones.

Reasons not to consume: This plant has resulted in an IgE anaphylaxis reaction in some individuals in a cross reaction with latex, legumes and figs. The proteins (lectins) are the source of the allergy, similar to what happens with prolamines in wheat. This plant has a high glycemic index and can be considered strongly inflammatory, like other grasses.

෫෫ ෫෫ ෫෫

Goosefoot -- *Family Amaranthaceae*: Plants like spinach, beet, sugar beet, chard, amaranth and quinoa are in this family. In this chapter, the focus will be on amaranth and quinoa. Both of these grains are native to the South American cultures.

High in Vitamins – B6, Folate, Thiamine, Choline, Betaine (high in quinoa).

High in Minerals – Calcium (high in amaranth), Copper, Iron, Magnesium, Manganese*, Phosphorus, Potassium, and Zinc.

Amino Acids Completeness – Goosefoot family members have a complete amino acid profile.

Consumption Profile	Amaranth uncooked 1 cup (193 g)	Quinoa uncooked 1 cup (170g)
Protein	26.2 g	24.0 g
Fat	13.5 g	10.3 g
Carbohydrates	127.0 g	109.0 g
Fiber	12.9 g	11.9 g

Key Chemical components – Lutein + Zeaxanthin, Omega-3 & 6 Essential fatty acids, Phytosterols, Lysine, Oxalates/Oxalic Acid (in leaves and stems), Saponins (in quinoa).

Reasons to consume: These two pseudo grains contain the highest quantity of protein as compared to other grasses. Their protein structure is complete to support our dietary needs. Their high fiber per serving is excellent for lowering cholesterol and supporting digestive health.

Reasons not to consume: High glycemic foods; strongly inflammatory especially for those with pre-existing arthritic/gout/rheumatoid conditions.

Food Combination – GRASSES & GRAINS

Grasses and grains in their minimally processed form take longer to digest as compared to other food families – between 2 and 3 hours. There is also phytic acid in these plants which have been known to inhibit digestion by blocking some of the enzymes necessary (pepsin, trypsin) to make the nutrients of these seeds accessible. In highly processed form, grains have minimal nutrients to digest and their time to break down is significantly reduced. That can lead to the empty caloric consumption and feeling hungry sooner.

Additionally, specific food combinations during meals increase the risk of reactivity. You may not have a reaction to either substance when eaten independently, however when combined, you may get an allergic or sensitivity reaction. The following combinations are considered risky for the Grasses & Grains Families:

– Corn with banana, dates or raisins
– Cane Sugar with orange
– Wheat with tea

The following plants and/or animals were evaluated to combine with grasses & grains to support optimal digestion:

Excellent – Green and low starch vegetables
Good – Fats & oils, mild starchy vegetables
Poor – Melons, fruits, animal proteins, nuts and seeds

Pollen interactions when consuming grasses & grains

Some folks have traditional IgE allergies from grasses. For example, ragweed (hay fever) in the Summer and Fall.. So, to consume a plant which you are allergic to seems counterproductive, right? Dr. Jacqueline Krohn and other physicians have documented examples of inhaling specific pollens which exacerbate allergic or sensitive reaction to foods consumed.

Pollen	Food Family/Members
Non food oriented Grass Pollens, Pecan Pollen, and Hickory Pollen	*Poaceae – Grass/Grains*

Blood Type Impacts

Dr. Peter D'Adamo has documented reactions of foods to people's health, based their on blood type in *Eat Right for your Type*. If you follow the specifics below for A or B blood types and still have issues, you may be a mixed blood type (part A or B and part O). Please refer to the Let's Get Started section to review for more information about mixed blood types. It would be best to evaluate both blood types' food specifics and see where your reactions lie.

Grasses/Grains to Avoid by Blood Type			
O	A	B	AB
Corn/Popcorn	Teff	Amaranth	Buckwheat/Kasha
Couscous (Cracked Wheat)	Wheat (Berry)	Barley	Corn/Popcorn
Gluten Flour	Wheat (Bran)	Buckwheat/Kasha	Kamut
Graham Flour	Wheat (Durum Flour products)	Corn/Popcorn	Soba Noodles (100% Buckwheat)
Wheat (Berry)	Wheat (Germ)	Couscous (Cracked Wheat)	Teff
Wheat (Bran)	Wheat (Whole Wheat Products)	Gluten Flour	
Wheat (Bulgur)		Kamut	
Wheat (Durum Flour products)		Rice (Wild)	
Wheat (Germ)		Rye Flour	
Wheat (Gluten Flour Products)		Rye/100% Rye Bread	
Wheat (Refined/Un/Bleached)		Teff	
Wheat (Semolina Flour Products)		Wheat (Berry)	
Wheat (White Flour Products)		Wheat (Bran)	
Wheat (Whole Wheat Products)		Wheat (Bulgur)	
Wheat Bread		Wheat (Durum Flour	

(Sprouted Commercial)		products)	
		Wheat (Germ)	
		Wheat (Gluten Flour Products)	
		Wheat (Whole Wheat Products)	

Grasses/Grains that are Beneficial by Blood Type			
O	A	B	AB
Buckwheat/Kasha	Amaranth	Millet	Buckwheat/Kasha
Rice (Cream of)	Buckwheat/Kasha	Oat Flour	Millet
Rice (puffed)/Rice Bran	Oat Flour	Oat/Oat Bran/Oatmeal	Oat Flour
Rice (White/Brown/Basmati) / Bread	Rice Cake/Flour	Rice (puffed)/Rice Bran	Oat/Oat Bran/Oatmeal
Rice Cake/Flour	Rye Flour	Spelt	Rice (Cream of)
	Soba Noodles (100% Buckwheat)		Rice (puffed)/Rice Bran
	Wheat Bread (Sprouted Commercial)		Rice (White/Brown/Basmati) / Bread
			Rice Cake/Flour
			Rye Flour
			Rye / 100% Rye Brea
			Spelt

All other grasses/grains not listed in tables have a neutral impact by blood types.

General Foodergies™ Issues

Grass family members/grains in general are suspect to one's health. Over 200 recent studies documented in PubMed and GreenMedInfo demonstrate and document how grass glutens impact our health. True, there are those few who do not have much, if any, reaction to the members of the Grass family at all.

Some individuals may have one or more of these below listed health conditions and illnesses and have not gotten any relief with basic diet/lifestyle changes. To help you support your conventional medical treatment, implementing a diet elimination and challenge test for this food family may help with:

- ADD or ADHD
- Autism
- Bipolar or Schizophrenia
- Brain fog
- Chronic anemia
- Chronic Fatigue Syndrome
- Colitis
- Crohn's disease
- Eczema
- Fibromyalgia
- Gall Bladder issues
- IBS
- Infertility or recurrent miscarriage
- Low thyroid (Hypothyroid)
- Lupus
- Migraine Headaches
- Multiple Sclerosis
- Osteoarthritis
- Osteoporosis
- Psoriasis
- Restless Legs Syndrome
- Rheumatoid Arthritis
- Scleroderma
- Sleep Apnea
- Those who suffer from chronic intestinal problems
- Type I or II diabetes

5 ANIMAL PROTEINS & DAIRY

From our earliest beginnings of mankind – we were hunters and gatherers. There were many periods of evolution before we learned animal husbandry – the art of domesticating animals for personal and eventually commercial food consumption. Today animal proteins and their derivatives have strayed far from their meager beginnings and we are not sure what is really in our meat, fish and dairy any more.

When it comes to consuming animal based proteins, there are many issues with their source, the treatment and commercialism of the animal, the ethics, and the quality and health of these creatures. For the sake of objectivity and scientific information sharing, the animal families' details are for commercially available proteins found in butcher shops, fish markets, grocery stores and farm markets.

I have a strong opinion on the quality and ethical treatment of animals produced for consumption. I have had periods of 50%-50% plant/animal consumption and been all the way to vegetarian/bordering vegan in my life time. Presently, I am an omnivore who eats 80% plants and 20% animal proteins, and have been for the last 3.5 years. I respect and give thanks to those who raise those animals in a compassionate, healthy and ethical way and waste nothing of their herds, flocks and stock. As a society of excess, one must be reminded that more is not always better and protein variety in our diets is the best option for our health.

Dairy Group:
- Cow's milk and all foods derived from cow's milk
  - Cheese, cottage cheese
  - Yogurt, kefir
  - Butter, ghee
- Eggs, (hen/chicken, duck, quail, ostrich)
- Goat's milk and all foods derived from goat's milk
  - Cheese
  - Yogurt
- Sheep's milk

Note: Milk replacements from nuts (almond milk, cashew milk), grains (rice milk, hemp milk, and oat milk), seeds (sunflower milk) or legumes (soy milk) are for those who have animal milk protein / sugar digestive issues/allergies. The best version of these milks are the no sugar added ones – you have to carefully check the ingredients and profile as some have over 10g of carbohydrate per 8 oz serving. Those carbohydrates are sugar based more than the source of the milk. Look for the unsweetened versions.

High in Vitamins – Vitamin A (butter and egg yolks) and D (milk, kefir, egg yolks). Also Folate, B12, Riboflavin and Pantothenic Acid though not in overwhelming quantities.

High in Minerals – Selenium is present in eggs. Calcium is present in cheeses and kefir. Phosphorus is present in egg yolks and cheese.

Amino Acids Completeness – Most dairy group members have a complete amino acid profile, with the exception of cow's milk; with milk other additional proteins need to be consumed to support necessary amino acid requirements in your diet.

Consumption Profile	Cow's Milk 3.25% 1 cup (244g)	Eggs, Chicken 1 Large Egg, Raw (50 g)	Goat Cheese 1 oz soft (28g)
Protein	7.9 g	6.3 g	5.2 g
Fat	7.9 g	5.0 g	5.9 g
Carbohydrates	12.8g	0.0 g	0.2 g
Fiber	0.0 g	4.0 g	0.0 g

Consumption Profile	Butter No salt 1 cup (227 g)	Cheddar Cheese 1 cup cubed (132 g)	Kefir plain unsweetened 1 Cup (180 g)
Protein	1.9 g	32.9 g	14.0 g
Fat	184.0 g	43.7 g	2.0 g
Carbohydrates	0.1 g	1.7 g	25.0 g
Fiber	0.0 g	0.0 g	3.0 g

Consumption Profile	Egg Whites (Chicken) 1 cup raw (243 g)	Egg Yolk (Chicken) 1 cup raw (243g)
Protein	26.5 g	38.5 g
Fat	0.4 g	64.5 g
Carbohydrates	1.8 g	8.7 g
Fiber	0.0 g	0.0 g

Key Chemical components – Members of the Dairy family have a natural opiate in them – casomorphin (part of the casinate – milk protein compound) – which is one of the reasons dairy can be "comforting" and addicting. Eggs have arachidonic acid and cholesterol.

Reasons to consume: The protein amounts found in dairy are most beneficial to us when we are young and maturing. Consuming fermented milk products like yogurt and kefir are beneficial to support our digestive and immune balance. Eggs are a complete protein source which is consumed by some vegetarians for their B12 component. A strictly plant-based diet lacks this crucial nutrient.

Reasons not to consume: Dairy based products are documented to precipitate irritation of the digestive tract especially with those folks who may have lactose intolerance. Lactose intolerance is a condition where the intestines do not have the ability to break down the milk sugar (lactose) in the dairy. Additionally, folks have milk protein allergies as well. Casein is the milk protein component that is extracted and used to support "non-dairy" products (non-lactose) in the form of sodium caseinate.

Eggs are one of the sensitive seven foods that are known to be the source of food intolerances and allergies. Folks can be sensitive to the albumin, the protein found in the white of the egg. or the arachidonic acid found in the yolk, or both. Eggs, like dairy products, are found in many processed products in various forms and usually found with gluten/grain based products – batters, cookies, breads and cakes.

Commercially made milk replacements with nuts, soy or grains (rice, hemp, and oat) have Carrageenan in them to facilitate emulsification and thickening of the nut, soy or grain particulates with the water. Numerous studies demonstrate that this algae derivative can be the source of respiratory and gastrointestinal inflammation. As with all things, moderation is key. Some of the sensitivities or intolerance symptoms you may have could go back this natural sourced additive.

Animal Meats

Cattle -- *Family Bovidae*. One of the earliest domesticated animals for human consumption were members of these animal family. Key members of this family are beef, goat, and lamb. In some countries, the only their part of the animal consumed is its milk.

High in Vitamins – Niacin, B6, B12, Riboflavin – especially high in the grass fed animals.

High in Minerals – Selenium, Phosphorus, Iron and Zinc.

Amino Acids Completeness – Beef family members have a complete amino acid profile.

Consumption Profile	Beef Grass Fed strip steak lean – raw (214 g)	Goat, raw (100 g)	Lamb, raw kabob (100 g)
Protein	49.4 g	93.4 g	20.2 g
Fat	5.8 g	10.5 g	5.3 g
Carbohydrates	0.0 g	0.0 g	0.0 g
Fiber	0.0 g	0.0 g	0.0 g

Key Chemical components – Members of the beef family have cholesterol as well as an excellent balance of protein amino acids.

Reasons to consume: For those who consume meat (regardless of the amount of sterols in the form of cholesterol) there are very few members of the food families as a whole which are as protein complete. When the animals are humanely treated, grass and pasture fed as they were originally, it can be one of the best sources of food.

Reasons not to consume: Commercial produced beef family members are subjected to unhealthy practices for "domestication." These animals are fed foods that are not part of their normal diet, changing the chemistry of the resultant proteins we end up consuming. Additionally, due to the poor sanitary conditions, these animals are supplemented with more medicines than the average human takes. These hormones and antibiotics are meant to keep them from getting sick while growing faster than nature intended.

There are other than humane reasons not to consume animals. It is due to the economies of cost to produce this level of protein: more money per acre to grow the feed, the transportation costs, on top of the medicine costs certainly has a bigger ecological and economic impact in the long run. The needs for humans to stay healthy with proteins can be mostly supported through different sources – mostly plants and then add some eggs to get the missing B12.

CB CB CB

Deer -- *Family Cervidae*: Deer (Venison) – It is one of the earliest meats available to eat back in the Paleolithic days. Today it is no longer a rare game meat to eat. It is much more widely consumed and is a great non-beef option.

High in Vitamins – Thiamine and B12.

High in Minerals – Zinc, Iron and Phosphorus.

Amino Acids Completeness – Deer has a complete amino acid profile; no other proteins are needed to support the necessary amino acid requirements in your diet.

Consumption Profile	Deer, Ground raw (100 g)
Protein	21.8 g
Fat	7.1 g
Carbohydrates	0.0 g
Fiber	0.0 g

Key Chemical components – Purines.

Reasons to consume: Lean lower fat "red" meat compared to beef; excellent balance of amino acids.

Reasons not to consume: Women and children should not eat the meat of these animals which was killed with lead bullets. Look for meat that was bow-hunted, if possible. The lead will leach through to the meat and when consumed, can build up in the body.

There is a current epidemic with deer here in the United States called Chronic Wasting Disease. It is a neurological disease in those animals and the concern is that is may spread to humans. However, there has been no documented proof of spreading or it being passed to humans through consumption of deer meat.

Also the natural occurrence of purines in the meat makes this a questionable choice for those suffering with gout or other rheumatic conditions.

CB CB CB

Pig -- *Family Suidae.* Pork is the key member of this family. Its two most commonly consumed "'y-products" are ham and bacon. This domesticated swine has an interesting consumption history. Members of certain religions forbid the consumption of this animal due to its unhygienic practices. With the "going to cleaner and healthier" methods of farming, pastured and hygienic raised pork has elevated the quality and safety of this animal product.

High in Vitamins – Thiamine, B6.

High in Minerals – Sodium, Selenium, and Phosphorus.

Amino Acids Completeness – Pork family has a complete amino acid profile.

Consumption Profile	Pork Fresh, raw carcass lean & fat (100 g)	Ham (Cured) 4 oz raw, center sliced cured (113 g)	Bacon (Cured) Raw 1 oz (28 g)
Protein	13.9 g	31.4 g	3.2 g
Fat	35.1 g	9.4 g	12.6 g
Carbohydrates	0.0 g	0.3 g	0.2 g
Fiber	0.0 g	0.0 g	0.0 g

Key Chemical components – Omega-6, Cholesterol.

Reasons to consume: Leaner cuts of meat with fewer grams of fat per serving which is comparable to the Galliformes family.

Reasons not to consume: Pork family members are naturally high in Sodium, even without preserving/curing with nitrates. Bacon still has cholesterol though not as much as ham or pork. Pork and ham levels of cholesterol are considered high for an animal product.

෪ ෪ ෪

Poultry -- *Order Galliformes:* This family speaks for itself. This is one of the most consumed animal proteins, next to ***Bovidae.***

- Family Anatidae – Duck: Duck and Goose
- Subfamily Family Phasianinae - Pheasant: Chicken, Cornish Hen
- Subfamily Family Tetraoninae – Grouse: Turkey

High in Vitamins – Niacin, Thiamine, Riboflavin, B6, Choline, Betaine.

High in Minerals – Selenium, Phosphorus, Iron, Copper.

Amino Acids Completeness – Poultry family members have a complete amino acid profile; no other proteins need to be consumed to support the necessary amino acid requirements in your diet.

Consumption Profile	Duck Raw Wild 1 lb (239 g)	Chicken 1lb raw skin and meat (276 g)	Turkey 1lb raw skin and meat (332 g)
Protein	41.6 g	51.3 g	67.8 g
Fat	36.3 g	41.6 g	26.6 g
Carbohydrates	0.0 g	0.0 g	0.0 g
Fiber	0.0 g	0.0 g	0.0 g

Key Chemical components – Omega-3 and 6: Omega-6 higher than 3 and cholesterol.

Reasons to consume: Leaner cuts of meat with fewer grams of fat per serving which is comparable to the Suidae family. There are more farms and organizations changing the way they cultivate their poultry. These new organic and pastured versions are becoming more accessible and mainstream for purchase. The nutrient content of these options can be noticeably higher based on the methods of farming.

Reasons not to consume: There are concerns with the commercially produced poultry stemming from their diet and farming conditions. This is no different than with pork or beef. Grass fed or pastured chickens allowed to feed as nature intended are healthier. However, the cost to raise and maintain chicken production in that fashion is still more expensive. Even organic farming has aspects of both practices which may produce a reasonable product.

Also, there is concern for *Salmonella* (food poisoning) as with all raw meat products and *Campylobacter* (a chicken specific bacterium). The *Salmonella* concern is mitigated using proper food handling, cooking and storing techniques. The issue with *Campylobacter* is that the bacterium is becoming resistant to the antibiotics that are used to treat the chickens. There are *fluoroquinolones (antibiotics)* that are sold to treat animals, and other forms are the leading treatment for humans who get food poisoning from that chicken bacterium. The mitigation for the *Campylobacter* is to eat Organic / Pastured chickens that would not be exposed to those antibiotics.

Seafood and Fish

Bony Fishes -- *Phylum Actinopterygii*: If early man did not hunt with his gathering, he fished. Harvesting from the sea is not unlike harvesting from a garden; there are water and nets involved. As far as animal proteins go, the bony fishes hold some of the best balances of animal proteins and essential fatty acids for our best health. Some of the commonly consumed members are listed below. For a more complete list, please refer back to Chapter 3 to the Food Family Summary.

- Flounder: Sole
- Mackerel: Mackerel, Tuna
- Cod: Cod (Scrod)
- Herring: Sardine
- Salmon: Salmon
- Sea Bass: Sea Bass
- Pike: Whitefish
- Catfish: Lake Catfish

High in Vitamins – B6, Niacin, B12. Some fish have higher Vitamin D due to the smaller fine bone content (mackerel, sardine, and sole). Also Choline and Betaine is found in these fishes.

High in Minerals – Selenium, Phosphorus (at varying levels).

Amino Acids Completeness – Bony fishes have a complete amino acid profile These members have the highest concentration of the key amino acids of any food family – flora or fauna.

Consumption Profile	Tuna fresh Bluefin raw 3 oz (85 g)	Salmon*** Wild Coho ½ Fillet (196 g)	Cod, Atlantic Raw fillet (231 g)
Protein	19.8 g	42.8 g	41.1 g
Fat	4.2 g	11.7 g	1.5 g
Carbohydrates	0.0 g	0.0 g	0.0 g
Fiber	0.0 g	0.0 g	0.0 g

Consumption Profile	Mackerel Atlantic Raw fillet (112 g)	Sardine Atlantic in Oil with Bone 1 cup drained (115 g)	Sole Raw fillet (163 g)
Protein	20.8 g	36.7 g	30.7 g
Fat	15.6 g	17.1 g	1.9 g
Carbohydrates	0.0 g	0.0 g	0.0 g
Fiber	0.0 g	0.0 g	0.0 g

Consumption Profile	Sea Bass Raw fillet (129 g)	Catfish, Wild Raw fillet (159 g)	Whitefish Raw fillet (198 g)
Protein	23.8 g	26.0 g	37.8 g
Fat	2.6 g	4.5 g	11.6 g
Carbohydrates	0.0 g	0.0 g	0.0 g
Fiber	0.0 g	0.0 g	0.0 g

*** *This fish is the most nutrient healthy of its peers – Atlantic versus Pacific, farmed versus wild caught.*

Key Chemical components – High Omega-3 and 6 proportions. Cholesterol more prevalent in Whitefish, Sardines, and Salmon.

Reasons to consume: Wild caught fish have 30% more vitamins and minerals than their farm raised siblings. Even the Omega-3 to Omega-6 ratios are higher (more 3 than 6 more significantly) with wild versus farm raised fish. This is most likely due to the diet fed to the farm raised fish. Farm raised fish are not always being fed like they would be in the wild. This leads to changes in the quality of the protein being formed. Remember what THEY eat becomes what WE eat, transformed.

Reasons not to consume: Farm raised fish which are raised on corn and soy by products are not being fed the proper diet to ensure normal genetic expression.

There is concern for wild caught fish due to the presence of heavy metals and pesticides (Mercury, Lead, and Phthalates). Our oceans and rivers are not as clean as they used to be. Please take that into account when consuming large quantities of fish on a consistent basis.

Also there are folks who have allergies due to a parasite that is commonly found in the fish. This parasite, Anisakis, is not known for causing anaphylaxis, however it does produce a traditional mild allergic response.

Additionally, individuals may suffer from Histamine Fish Poisoning which can produce similar symptoms to an allergic attack; nausea, vomiting, diarrhea, hives, itching, rash and a burning sensation in the mouth (similar to Oral Allergy Syndrome). Symptoms can start a few minutes after you eat the fish, and last up to 24 hours This is the result of a bacteria found in the fish which produces histadine in strong concentration. The histadine is converted into histamine and produces the reaction. This condition is most commonly found in the Scombroid group of fishes.

ᴄꙅ　ᴄꙅ　ᴄꙅ

Phylum Crustacea - Crustacean: Crab, Shrimp, Lobster are the three most commonly consumed members of this food family. Bottom dwellers and scavengers by nature, these creatures do a great deal of the clean up and microbiological sprucing of the sea floor and deep waters.

High in Vitamins – Shrimp has some Vitamin D and Choline. Others not much if any.

High in Minerals – Sodium, Selenium, Copper and Zinc.

Amino Acids Completeness – Crustaceans have a complete amino acid profile; no other proteins need to be consumed to support the necessary amino acid requirements in your diet.

Consumption Profile	Crab King raw (172 g)	Lobster 1 Whole Atlantic raw (150 g)	Shrimp, raw (100 g)
Protein	31.5 g	28.2 g	20.3 g
Fat	1.0 g	1.3 g	1.7 g
Carbohydrates	0.0 g	0.7 g	0.9 g
Fiber	0.0 g	0.0 g	0.0 g

Key Chemical components – Iodine.

Reasons to consume: Low in cholesterol. These food family members are considered anti-inflammatory foods.

Reasons not to consume: Naturally high in sodium and need to watch for those with high blood pressure. Additionally, there are a significant number of people who have allergies to these creatures. It could be the fact that they eat detritus (similar to mollusk) and that become the "protein" we eat from them. Also, it could be the naturally high levels of Iodine or chitin in their bodies that folks react to. Those elements are bound to the "flesh" and for some that is the real trigger, not the animal itself.

ଓଷ ଓଷ ଓଷ

Phylum Mollusca - Mollusk: This family of ocean creatures is one of the more common allergic/sensitive families in the animal kingdom. Their habitat is one of being in collectives and performing mass filtering and clearing of areas of phytoplankton and microbes. Some of the most popularly consumed members are listed here:

– Gastropods: Snails
– Cephalopods: Squid
– Pelecycpods: Clam, Oyster, Scallop, Mussel

High in Vitamins – B12.

High in Minerals – Iron, Selenium, Zinc, Manganese, Copper.

Amino Acids Completeness – Most mollusks have a complete amino acid profile Snails are the exception as they need additional proteins to make a complete protein profile.

Consumption Profile	Clams 1 cup raw (227 g)	Oysters Pacific raw 1 med (50 g)	Mussels Blue, raw 1 cup (150 g)
Protein	29.0 g	4.7 g	17.9 g
Fat	2.2 g	1.1 g	3.4 g
Carbohydrates	5.8 g	2.5 g	5.6 g
Fiber	0.0 g	0.0 g	0.0 g

Consumption Profile	Squid raw (100 g)	Scallops raw (100 g)	Snails raw 1 oz (28 g)
Protein	15.6 g	16.8 g	4.5 g
Fat	1.4 g	0.8 g	0.4 g
Carbohydrates	3.1 g	2.4 g	0.6 g
Fiber	0.0 g	0.0 g	0.0 g

Key Chemical components – Omega-3 & Omega-6

Reasons to consume: Most natural concentration of B12 compared to land animals.

Reasons not to consume: Same reasons as with Crustaceans. Their extensive filtering system allows them to consume some less than appealing substances. In return, they produce a small concentrated protein for our consumption. From an economic perspective, extensive farming and the needs for repopulation due to over-harvesting can take its toll on the quality of this protein. These animals are highly susceptibility to toxic algae blooms which makes these family members be in short supply and high demand. Also, this food family is susceptible to domoic acid which is produced by the microscopic algae they filter. Cooking does not eliminate this or other poisonous substances.

Food Combination – ANIMAL PROTEINS & DAIRY

The best form of dairy to consume is raw, unpasteurized from grass-fed organic sources, naturally cultured like kefir/homemade yogurt, or organic non-dairy products (nut, grass, seed milks).

Eggs are one of those foods where minimally processed is best. If you are capable of consuming these foods, they should be from free range and cage free chickens. cooking eggs in scrambled form releases too much arachidonic acid and is not the best way to consume them.

The optimal animal proteins to consume are from wild caught, grass fed, humanely treated/free range/pastured environments. There are still so many issues with farm raised/commercially raised and processed meats and fishes; non-native or typical diets are fed those animals to increase their maturity and ability to be mass produced, and their living conditions being confining and not like their natural environment. It is not natural for fish to be fed corn, much less other animals (especially the mass manipulated GMO corn produced today).

Fish can be consumed raw in the form of sushi and sashimi, however it is not considered healthy as the proteins can be polluted with bacteria or parasites. That is why sushi is consumed with soy sauce, ginger and wasabi so that it attempts to neutralize and decontaminate what is being consumed.

Animal proteins are created like our cells in our bodies are created – by what they eat! If they eat GMO, their cells are responding to the mutated sources and producing insufficient structures. If they eat 'garbage' their cells are deficient or even damaged or mutated; what they eat – you end up eating.

Remember a cow has multiple stomachs and chews its food a lot, even more than we do. It is in their nature to ensure the enzymes are released and the multiple stomachs can be more efficient in digestion. We have only one stomach and we sure put a wider variety of foods into it.

Note for eating – chew your food until almost liquid and your digestion will thank you.

When animal proteins are prominent in a full sized meal, it can take *longer* (between 3 and 4 hours) for the stomach to empty due to the extra digestion processing. Proteins are difficult to break down just like fats and with out sufficient stomach acids and enzymes it just takes longer.

Additionally, specific food combinations during meals increase the risk of reactivity. You may not have a reaction to either substance when eaten independently, however when combined you may get an allergic or sensitivity reaction. The following combinations are considered risky for the Animal Protein & Dairy families:

- Egg & apple
- Beef & yeast
- Pork & black pepper
- Chicken & pork
- Milk & mint
- Milk & chocolate

The following plants and/or animals are evaluated to combine with Animal Proteins & Dairy:

Excellent – Soybeans, non starchy vegetables
Good – Nuts and Seeds, mildly starchy vegetables
Poor – Grasses & grains, most legumes, oils & fats, gourds

Pollen interactions when consuming Animal Proteins & Dairy

Can inhaling specific pollens exacerbate allergic or sensitive reaction to foods consumed? Additionally, can having a specific condition increase the sensitivity or reactions to food? Dr. Jacqueline Krohn and other physicians have documented examples of these occurrences.

Pollen	Food Family/Members
Dust	Mollusca – Shellfish
Cedar Pollen, Juniper Pollen	Bovidae - Beef
Elm Pollen, Oak Pollen, Ragweed Pollen and Viral Infections	Dairy
Poison Ivy	Suidae - Pork

Blood Type Impacts

To reiterate Dr. Peter D'Adamo has documented reactions of foods to health based on blood type in *Eat Right for your Type*. If you follow the specifics below for A or B blood types and still have issues, you may be a mixed blood type (part A or B and part O). Please refer to the Let's Get Started section to review for more information about mixed blood types. It would be best to evaluate both blood types' food specifics and see where your reactions lie.

Dairy** to Avoid by Blood Type			
O	A	B	AB
American Cheese	American Cheese	American Cheese	American Cheese
Blue Cheese	Blue Cheese	Blue Cheese	Blue Cheese
Brie Cheese	Brie Cheese	Ice Cream	Brie Cheese
Buttermilk	Butter	String Cheese	Butter
Camembert Cheese	Buttermilk		Buttermilk
Casein/Caseinate	Camembert Cheese		Camembert Cheese
Cheddar Cheese	Casein/Caseinate		Half & Half
Colby Cheese	Cheddar Cheese		Ice Cream
Cottage Cheese	Colby Cheese		Milk (Whole-Cow)
Cream Cheese	Cottage Cheese		Parmesan Cheese
Edam Cheese	Cream Cheese		Provolone Cheese
Emmenthal Cheese	Edam Cheese		Sherbet
Goat Cheese	Emmenthal Cheese		
Gouda Cheese	Gouda Cheese		
Gruyere Cheese	Gruyere Cheese		
Half & Half	Half & Half		
Ice Cream	Ice Cream		
Jarlsberg Cheese	Jarlsberg Cheese		
Kefir	Monterey Jack		
Milk – Skim or 2% (Cow)	Muenster Cheese		
Milk – Whole (Cow)	Neufchatel Cheese		
Milk (Goat)	Paneer		
Monterey Jack	Parmesan Cheese		
Muenster Cheese	Provolone Cheese		
Neufchatel Cheese	Quark Cheese		
Paneer	Sherbet		
Parmesan Cheese	String Cheese		

Provolone Cheese	Swiss Cheese		
Ricotta Cheese	Whey/Whey Protein Supplement		
Sherbet			
Sour Cream (low/non-fat)			
String Cheese			
Swiss Cheese			
Whey/Whey Protein Supplement			

*** Includes non animal protein milk substitutes*

Dairy** that are Beneficial by Blood Type			
O	A	B	AB
Rice Milk	Kefir	Cottage Cheese	Cottage Cheese
	Milk (Goat)	Farmer Cheese	Egg Whites (Albumin)
	Mozzarella Cheese	Feta Cheese	Farmer Cheese
	Ricotta Cheese	Goat Cheese	Feta Cheese
	Soy Cheese	Kefir	Goat Cheese
	Soy Milk	Milk (Skim or 2% - Cow)	Kefir
		Milk (Goat)	Milk (Goat)
		Paneer	Mozzarella Cheese
		Rice Milk	Rice Milk
		Ricotta Cheese	Ricotta Cheese
		Yogurt	Sour Cream (low/non-fat)
			Yogurt

*** Includes non animal protein milk substitutes*

Meats to Avoid by Blood Type			
O	A	B	AB
Bacon/Ham/Pork	Bacon/Ham/Pork	Bacon/Ham/Pork	Bacon/Ham/Pork
Goose	Beef	Chicken	Beef
	Buffalo	Cornish Hens	Buffalo
	Duck	Duck	Chicken
	Goat	Goose	Cornish Hens
	Goose	Partridge	Duck
	Lamb	Quail	Goat
	Mutton		Goose
	Pheasant		Partridge
	Rabbit		Quail
	Veal		Veal
	Venison		Venison

Meats that are Beneficial by Blood Type

O	A (only occasionally)	B	AB
Beef	Chicken	Lamb	Lamb
Buffalo	Cornish Hens	Mutton	Mutton
Lamb	Turkey	Rabbit	Rabbit
Mutton		Venison	Turkey
Turkey			
Veal			
Venison			

Fish/Shellfish to Avoid by Blood Type

O	A	B	AB
Barracuda	Anchovy	Anchovy	Anchovy
Catfish	Barracuda	Barracuda	Barracuda
Caviar	Bass – Bluegill	Bass – Bluegill	Bass – Bluegill
Conch	Bass – Striped	Bass – Sea	Bass – Sea
Herring/Kippers - Pickled	Beluga	Bass – Striped	Bass – Striped
Lox	Bluefish	Beluga	Beluga
Octopus	Catfish	Clam	Clam
	Caviar	Conch	Conch
	Clam	Crab	Crab
	Conch	Crab – Horseshoe	Crab – Horseshoe
	Crab	Crawfish/Crayfish	Crawfish/Crayfish
	Crawfish/Crayfish	Eel	Eel
	Eel	Lobster	Flounder
	Flounder	Lox	Gray Sole
	Gray Sole	Mussels	Haddock
	Grouper	Octopus	Hake
	Haddock	Oyster	Halibut
	Hake	Shrimp	Herring/Kippers – Pickled
	Halibut	Snail – Escargot	Lobster
	Herring/Kippers – Pickled	Yellowtail	Lox
	Lobster		Octopus
	Lox		Oyster
	Mussels		Shrimp
	Octopus		Sole
	Oyster		Yellowtail
	Scallop		
	Shad		

	Shrimp		
	Sole		
	Squid		
	Tilefish		

Fish/Shellfish that are Beneficial by Blood Type			
O	A	B	AB
Bass – Striped	Carp	Caviar	Cod
Bluefish	Cod	Cod	Flounder
Cod	Mackerel	Flounder	Grouper
Hake	Monkfish	Grouper	Haddock
Halibut	Perch – Silver	Haddock	Hake
Herring/Kippers (Fresh)	Perch – Yellow	Hake	Halibut
Mackerel	Pickerel	Halibut	Mackerel
Monkfish	Red Snapper	Mackerel	Mahi-Mahi
Perch (White)	Salmon – Wild	Mahi-Mahi	Monkfish
Perch (Yellow)	Sardine	Monkfish	Perch – Ocean
Pike	Snail - Escargot	Perch –Ocean	Pickerel
Red Snapper	Trout – Rainbow	Pickerel	Pike
Salmon – Wild	Trout – Sea	Pike	Porgy
Sardine	Whitefish	Porgy	Red Snapper
Shad		Salmon – Wild	Sailfish
Smelt		Sardine	Sardine
Snapper		Shad	Shad
Sole		Sole	Snail – Escargot
Sturgeon		Sturgeon	Sturgeon
Swordfish		Trout – Sea	Trout – Rainbow
Tilefish			Trout – Sea
Trout – Rainbow			Tuna
Tuna			
Whitefish			
Yellowtail			

All other animal proteins and dairy not listed in tables have a neutral impact by blood types.

Note: Blood type B is the most tolerant of consuming Dairy group members; Blood type O is the least tolerant. Blood type O is the most tolerant of Animal Proteins; Blood Type A is the least tolerant. This is very much in line with the evolution of our blood types and the scope of the foods available to us at that time.

General Foodergies™ Issues

Animal food families are unrelated to each other. Being sensitive to beef is not going to make you sensitive to pork or fish. The animals which have the most inter-reactivity are in the fish/shellfish families. This would have to do with what those fish or shellfish eat. For example, shellfish sensitivity and allergies relate to the consumption of that protein and what makes it up. *Remember* – "you are what you eat" extends even to the animal families too. So, what do shrimp, lobster, clams or scallops eat ? Detritus and other sea animal feces and microorganisms. To extend that definition – would you want to eat a protein that was fed on dead, decaying material, feces and microbes? It would be a logical progression to assume those toxins that were created, left over or present in that "fuel" for the shellfish would extend into the protein we would consume. Certain species of shellfish – clams, oysters and mussels - filter, strip and take only what was needed to be consumed and excrete the rest. Those creatures may have a less toxic profile for allergies and sensitivities compared to a similar mollusk – scallops. The same would go for the fish families – what they eat impacts the kind of protein that is created in their bodies and what we end up consuming. For example, catfish also are bottom dwellers and sift through detritus as well. It may be tasty, however it may not be as healthy as other fish.

There are individuals who have issues consuming specific animal proteins for health reasons e.g., primary hypertension or gout. There are options with animal proteins and dairy that is supportive and corrective to one's health. One specific case is a client of mine who has primary hypertension. His blood pressure on the standard American diet was over 170/130. He considered himself healthier than most; not overweight, working out 4-5 times a week, lots of water and balanced meals. However his blood pressure would spike consistently into dangerously high ranges. We worked together on a Food Friendly (no Foodergies™) plan consisting of a lacto-ovo (specific dairy and egg) vegetarian food members. Within a week he was able to lower his blood pressure to 120/80 and maintain it. When he strays from the plan, he has times where he spikes out of range. Through the education on food families and his specific Foodergies™, he knows what it will take to restore it on his own. He states he can feel the difference within hours of correcting his food behavior.

6 LEGUMES

This food family is known for being the most digestively discomforting on an everyday basis. Legumes also known as "Beans" composed the majority of the protein in the vegetarian and vegan diet landscape. This is the third largest land plant family (first is Orchids (Orchidaceae), second is the Daisy (Asteraceae)).

Members of Family Fabaceae / Leguminosae – There are quite a few groups of legumes (bean and pea). Legumes have been a food source since 6000 BC, where they were a protein replacement when animal protein was scarce. Each bullet delineates similar species/subfamilies of legumes:

- Soybean
- Haricot Beans (Phaseolus) – Green Bean (Snap Bean), Lima Bean, Butter Bean, Common Bean, Black Bean, Kidney Bean, Red Bean, White Bean (Cannellini or Navy Bean), Cranberry Bean, Pinto Bean
- Peas – Snow Pea, Sugar Snap Pea, Common Pea (Mangetout Peas – eaten whole with pod before maturity)
- Chickpeas
- Peanut
- Adzuki (Azuki) bean, Black Eyed Pea, Mung Bean
- Broad Bean, Fava Bean, Lentil
- Carob
- Jicama

High in Vitamins – Peanuts are high in Niacin, Thiamine and Folate. Adzuki bean are high in Folate. Jicama is a reasonable source of Vitamin C. Chickpeas are high in Folate, Thiamine and B6. Lentils are high in Folate and Thiamine. Soybean has high levels of Folate, Vitamin K, Thiamine and Riboflavin. Green Peas have high Vitamin C and K. Most of the Haricot bean group has high Folate and Thiamine.

High in Minerals – Peanuts are high in Manganese, Magnesium, Phosphorus and Copper. Adzuki bean are high in Manganese. Chickpeas are high in Manganese, Copper, Phosphorus, and Iron. Lentils are high in Manganese, Phosphorus, Iron and Zinc. Mature soybeans have high Manganese, Iron, Copper, Phosphorus, Magnesium, and Potassium. Most of the Haricot bean group is high in Manganese, Magnesium, Potassium and Phosphorus.

Amino Acids Completeness – Most legumes do not have a complete amino acid profile to support necessary protein consumption in your diet. Chickpeas, Red Kidney Bean, Black Bean, White (Haricot/Navy) Beans and Mature Soybeans (not green) have a complete amino acid profile.

Consumption Profile	Peas, Green raw (145 g)	Haricot Beans (group) 1 cup (193 g)	Adzuki Bean – Boiled no salt 1 cup (230 g)
Protein	7.9 g	41.3 g	17.3 g
Fat	0.6 g	2.4 g	0.2 g
Carbohydrates	21.0 g	121.0 g	57.0 g
Fiber	7.4 g	29.9 g	16.8 g

Consumption Profile	Lentil – raw 1 cup (192g)	Soybean – Mature, raw 1 cup (186 g)	Peanuts - Dry Roasted no salt 1 cup (146g)
Protein	49.5 g	67.9 g	34.6 g
Fat	2.0 g	37.1 g	72.5 g

Carbohydrates	115.0 g	56.1 g	31.4 g
Fiber	58.6 g	17.3 g	11.7 g

Consumption Profile	Jicama – raw 1 cup sliced (120 g)	Carob – unsweetened candies (100 g)	Chickpeas – raw 1 cup (200 g)
Protein	0.9 g	8.1 g	38.6 g
Fat	0.1 g	31.4 g	12.1 g
Carbohydrates	10.6 g	56.3 g	121.0 g
Fiber	5.9 g	3.8 g	34.8 g

Key Chemical components – Nitrogen fixing in the roots – could be related to the "natural gas" release when being consumed.

Reasons to consume: High in fiber, great for lowering cholesterol and keeping digestion smooth. Kidney beans (Haricot) are known for supporting renal functions. According to the Doctrine of Signatures, these Beans help the healing process and kidney filtering processes.

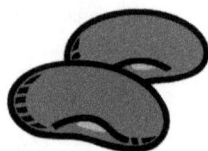

Reasons not to consume: Can be difficult to digest. Lectins which cause agglutination. Peanuts have really high Omega-6 to Omega-3 ratio.

Food Combination – LEGUMES

Legumes can be consumed raw or cooked; if dried to start, it is better for the legumes to be soaked between 4 hours and over night. Once the legumes are soaked, cooking them to break up the complex protein structures to make them easier to digest. When legumes are prominent in a full sized meal, it can take *longer* (between 3 and 4 hours) for the stomach to empty. These food family members require extra digestive effort on the proteins and complex carbohydrate structures.

The following plants and/or animals are evaluated to combine with Legumes:

Excellent – Non starchy vegetables, other starchy vegetables/potatoes (e.g. Gourd family), grasses & grains
Good – Mildly starchy vegetables, oils & fats
Poor – Animal & Dairy Family, soybeans***, fungi

*** *It is a different species which unique protein profile making it more complex to digest.*

Pollen interactions when consuming legumes

Can inhaling specific pollens exacerbate allergic or sensitive reaction to foods consumed? Additionally, can having a specific condition increase the sensitivity or reactions to food? Dr. Jacqueline Krohn and other physicians have documented examples of these occurrences.

Pollen	Food Family/Members
Grass Pollens	Fabaceae – Legumes
Mugwort Pollen	Peanuts
Birch Pollen	Fabaceae – Legumes

Blood Type Impacts

Dr. Peter D'Adamo is the Naturopathic specialist whose research on blood type food reactions is documented in his book, *Eat Right for your Type*. If you follow the specifics below for A or B blood types and still have issues, you may be a mixed blood type (part A or B and part O). Please refer to the Let's Get Started section to review for more information about mixed blood types. Review both blood types' food specifics and see where your reactions lie.

Legumes to Avoid by Blood Type			
O	A	B	AB
Copper Bean	Copper Beam	Adzuki Bean	Adzuki Bean
Kidney Bean	Garbanzo Bean	Black Bean	Black Bean
Lentil – Domestic	Kidney Bean	Black Eyed Pea	Black Eyed Pea
Lentil – Green	Lima Bean	Garbanzo Bean	Fava Bean
Lentil – Red	Navy Bean	Lentil – Domestic	Garbanzo Bean
Navy Bean	Red Bean	Lentil – Green	Kidney Bean
Tamarind	Tamarind	Lentil – Red	Lima Bean
		Mung Bean (Sprouts	Mung Bean (Sprouts)
		Pinto Bean	

Legumes that are Beneficial by Blood Type			
O	A	B	AB
Adzuki Bean	Adzuki Bean	Kidney Bean	Lentil – Green
Black Eyed Pea	Black Bean	Lima Bean	Navy Bean
Pinto Bean	Black Eyed Pea	Navy Bean	Pinto Bean
	Green Bean	Soybean	Red Bean
	Lentil – Domestic		Soybean
	Lentil – Green		
	Lentil – Red		
	Pinto Bean		
	Soybean		

All other legumes not listed in tables have a neutral impact by blood types.

There are cultural adjustments to this list that needs to be made based on geographic region and genetics. Certain blood types were raised on beans which according to the list may need to be avoided or had occasionally like on a rotation diet – e.g. O blood types from West Indies consuming red beans or kidney beans with their "Rice and peas."

General Foodergies™ Issues

Legumes have many benefits and drawbacks. For those who are peanut Allergic – IgE/Anaphylaxis – you have to be very careful of the legumes you consume or better yet avoid them all. Peanuts (a legume), as well as all shelled tree nuts, are susceptible to *Aflatoxin* – a deadly mycotoxin found in *Aspergillus flavus* and *Parasiticus* bacteria, which can make you very ill. The

Aflatoxin may be found in some processed peanut butters as well as in packaged shelled nuts.

At the end of the day, there are plenty of places to find vegetable protein without the digestive challenges and immune issues. Check out the Commonly Consumed Fruit & Vegetables chapter (Chapter 10) to find other plants which can fill in the gap that legumes leave.

7 NIGHTSHADES

With all the foods that we eat and the health problems we have, it is important to single out the Nightshade family of plants. Misunderstood, misinterpreted and overused, these plants have a significant impact on our diet and our health.

The family is named after its founding plant member, Belladonna – Solanum Nigrum, also known as Deadly Nightshade. Other plants were classified in this group – the Capsicum Peppers and Lycium species (Wolfberry – also known as Goji Berry). This was because of the similar chemical composition of their fruits and plant identification criteria (leaves, seed structure, flowers, etc.).

Early in our documented food consumption history, a ban of tomatoes took place. When the tomato plant was identified as part of the Deadly Nightshade family, folks thought it would be poisonous or as toxic as the primary plant in the family, Deadly Nightshade (Belladonna). For at least 400 years, folks did not consume or grow tomatoes for eating, just ornamentally. Once more investigation took place to differentiate these plants from its medicinal and toxic family member, tomatoes were consumed again. A similar story could be told about potatoes in the 15th century. Queen Elizabeth I was presented a gift of potatoes. Since they never had them before, they cooked everything – leaves, stems and the tubers and the members of the court got very ill so the plant was banned. Later the Queen bequeathed land for the growth of these plants so these foods could be fed to the oppressed Irish. Later when experience and subsequent education on how to consume these plants occurred, fewer people got sick. As a result, consumption of these plants during this impoverished time was key to communities' survival.

A little known fact about our friends the Nightshades is that they are naturally high in a trace mineral called Lithium. Elemental Lithium is found in the soil and enters these plants and fixates in the fruits/flesh. Commercial *Lithium carbonate* (a salt) is used to help mental health issues of bipolar disorder/mood swings. There was a woman on my project team at one of my software clients who used to say "If I don't get my daily potato fix, I am not a happy person". It was true, she was more irritable, easily confused, and more emotional when she did not have her potato a day – did not matter how, mashed, boiled or fried. This Lithium tie would be a "eureka" moment in my own personal dietary analysis.

There are other allergy and intolerance triggering chemicals in these plants – glycoalkaloids present in the top layers of the fruit/tubers close to the skin which have been documented to cause illness, neuralgia and digestive upset. So with this kind of bad press, why do we still consume these plants?

> *To think how many peppers I packed into my snacking diet as a child; the fresh garden Tomatoes, the homemade freshly made fried potatoes with ketchup* ☺ *- I sigh and shudder thinking what did to myself??? You never know about your genetics until you learn about it later in life. Hindsight is not 20/20 – more like a smack upside the head.*
>
> *Why does a mid 40 year old woman have arthritis of a 75 year old? My surgeon could not explain it. My first Rheumatologist said I was "genetically crunchy" and that was not enough of an explanation for me. My second Rheumatologist and myself are digging deeper into the WHY – and it has ties to my genetics as well as my diet. One of those components used to be the Nightshade family – and they are no longer in my diet and I will explain why it may also be something for you to evaluate as well.*

Members of Potato -- Family Solanaceae: Potato (white, red, blue and yellow), tomato, eggplant, peppers (bell, red, green, chile, cayenne, jalapeño), goji berry and tomatillo.

High in Vitamins – Potatoes, tomatoes, bell peppers and jalapeño peppers are a good source of Vitamin C. Goji berries are high in Vitamin C and Riboflavin. Red bell peppers have a high concentration of Vitamin A.

High in Minerals – Goji Berries are high in Iron and Selenium. Capsicum peppers are rich in Sulfur.

Amino Acids Completeness – Nightshade family members have an incomplete amino acid profile. Other additional protein sources are needed to complement and provide a complete amino acid profile.

Consumption Profile	Bell Pepper (red, yellow, green averaged) (100 g)	Potato, white – raw ½ Cup Diced (75 g)	Tomato (yellow, red, orange and green averaged) (100 g)
Protein	1.3 – 1.9 g green - yellow	1.3 g	1.3 – 2.2 g yellow – green
Fat	0.3 – 0.4 g	0.1 g	0.3 – 0.4 g
Carbohydrates	6.9 – 11.8 g green – yellow	12.8 g	4.1 – 9.2 g yellow - green
Fiber	1.7 – 3.1 g yellow - red	1.8 g	1.0 – 2.0 g yellow –green

Consumption Profile	Jalapeño Peppers – 1 cup sliced (90 g)	Eggplant – raw 1 Cup Cubed (82 g)	Tomatillo– ½ c chopped (66 g)
Protein	1.2 g	0.8 g	0.6 g
Fat	0.6 g	0.2 g	0.7 g
Carbohydrates	5.6 g	4.7 g	3.9 g
Fiber	2.5 g	2.8 g	1.3 g

Consumption Profile	Goji Berry – dried (100 g)
Protein	10.6 g
Fat	0.7 g
Carbohydrates	21.0 g
Fiber	4.7 g

Key Chemical components:

Component	Tomato (Red)	Potato	Tomatillo	Bell Pepper	Jalapeño Pepper	Goji Berry	Eggplant
Calcitriol	√	√					
Solanine	√	√	√	√	√	√	√
Chaconine		√					
Nicotine	√						√
Tomatine	√						
Lycopene	√					√	
Capsaicin					√		
Beta-carotene	√	√	√	√	√	√	√
Lutein	√	√	√	√	√	√	
Zeaxanthin	√	√	√	√	√	√	
polysaccharides (antioxidant)					√	√	
Beta sitosterol						√	

Reasons to consume: The wonderful myriad of phytonutrients available makes these plants a great choice to eat and cook with. Members of this family have anticancer, anti-cholesterol, antimicrobial, anti-inflammatory, anti-nocieceptive and antipyretic benefits. Lycopene has been shown to lower cancer risk in humans along with Beta-carotene. This red carotene has been shown to reduce chance of heart disease, prevent cataracts and macular degeneration. It is those antioxidant properties which neutralize the free radicals before they can do damage in the body. Research shows that tomatoes are supportive to the heart and blood. The Doctrine of Signatures demonstrates the similarities between our heart and the tomato; both have four chambers and have red pigment.

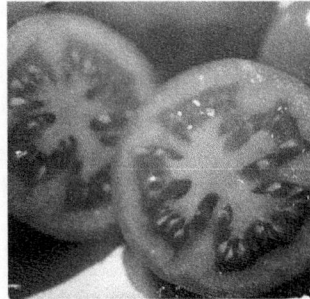

Skins of potatoes and eggplant have chlorogenic acid – a polyphenol that are shown to be preventative of cancer cell mutation. The flesh of a raw potato has protease inhibitors which are good for neutralizing viruses. Eggplants have anticonvulsant compounds of scopoletin and scoparone. Capsicum peppers have analgesic, antibacterial, anticancer, and antioxidant properties. Bell peppers have antioxidant and Salicylate properties.

Reasons not to consume: Even though the members of this family have beneficial properties, there are reactions that are coupled with those positive benefits. The key glycoalkaloid toxins of solanine, nicotine and have been known to cause skin irritation, inflammation and digestive disorders. Calcitriol (active form of Vitamin D) found in these plant family members may impact the ability of some individuals to process it without causing soft Calcium deposits.

Nightshades are one of the key families who trigger Oral Allergy Syndrome in some folks. Eggplant is one of the biggest culprits due to its high concentration of natural histamine. Tomatoes also do this, however it is more the acidity and the solanine/tomatine that is precipitating the reaction.

Food Combination – NIGHTSHADES

When Nightshades are prominent in a full sized meal, it can take *longer* (between 2 and 3 hours) for the stomach to empty due to the extra digestion processing. The only Nightshade which has food combining challenges is the potato, due to its starchy/carbohydrate heavy nature. Potatoes combined with animal or legume protein are not suggested due to the excess digestive workload they produce. Other Nightshades are considered non-starchy vegetables and can be combined with everything, except fruit. The tomatoes is the most acidic of the Nightshade family members and as a "fruit" should be consumed on its own.

The following plants and/or animals are evaluated to combine with Nightshades (except for potatoes):

Excellent – Animal & Dairy, mildly starchy vegetables, oils & fats, nuts & seeds, non starchy vegetables.
Good – Potatoes combine reasonably well with oils & fats, mildly starchy vegetables
Poor – Potatoes do not combine well with animal & dairy or fungi

Pollen interactions when consuming Nightshades

Can inhaling specific pollens exacerbate allergic or sensitive reaction to foods consumed? Additionally, can having a specific condition increase the sensitivity or reactions to food? Dr. Jacqueline Krohn and other physicians have documented examples of these occurrences:

Pollen	Food Family/Members
Birch, Sage and Mugwort Pollens	Solanaceae – Nightshades
Latex-Fruit Allergy Syndrome	Solanaceae – Nightshades

Blood Type Impacts

Dr. Peter D'Adamo has documented reactions of foods to health based on blood type in *Eat Right for your Type*. If you follow the specifics below for A or B blood types and still have issues, you may be a mixed blood type (part A or B and part O). Please refer to the Let's Get Started section to review for more information about mixed blood types. It would be best to evaluate both blood types' food specifics and see where your reactions lie.

Nightshades to Avoid by Blood Type			
O	A	B	AB
Eggplant	Eggplant	Tomato	Green/Yellow/Jalapeno Peppers
Potato (White, Red, Blue, Yellow)	Green/Yellow/Jalapeno Peppers		Cayenne Pepper
	Cayenne Pepper		
	Potato (White, Red, Blue, Yellow)		
	Tomato		

Nightshades that are Beneficial by Blood Type			
O	A	B	AB
Cayenne Pepper		Eggplant	Eggplant
		Green/Yellow/Jalapeno Peppers	
		Cayenne Pepper	

All other Nightshade family members not listed in tables have a neutral impact by blood types.

> *Goji Berries and Tomatillos are not rated on the traditional Eat Right 4 Your Type –*
> *they have been classified based on GenoType/SWAMI program.*

General Foodergies™ Issues

Nightshades are ones of those things you have to decide for yourself if you want to try removing it or not. Not many folks want to give up their mashed potatoes, their fresh garden tomatoes or hot sauce. It is suggested that if you are experiencing joint pain and aches and cannot figure out from where or why – eliminate them completely from your diet for at least 3 weeks. Not just cut back, just don't eat them and see how you feel without them. Then add each plant back every four days and see how you feel. It is strongly suggested to do a short cleanse before performing this evaluation due to the nature of the toxins and how they may be stored in the fat cells. Due to constraints and conditions in your life, it may not be possible to do.

If you do choose to consume members of this family, there are ways of lessening your exposure to the glycoalkaloids:

– Remember to consume these family members in their ripest forms; tomatoes when they are not green and potatoes that do not have any green tint to their skin.

– Keep potatoes in the cool and dark to retard the glycoalkaloid formation.

– Discard any potatoes that have sprouted eyes or have blemishes or rotted areas.

– Remember to discard leaves or stems and not consume from either plant (potato or tomato) as the concentration of the glycoalkaloid is at its highest and is considered toxic to consume.

For every study that says Nightshades are fine and the research shows there are not correlations, there are others which show issues with the glycoalkaloids and pain in mammals along with a lot of anecdotal statements. It is safe to say, if you have cut back on your Nightshades or eliminated them, then went back to eating them with no change in health, there is nothing to be concerned about. The positive nutrients and concentration of Lithium alone makes this a wonderful plant family despite its name.

For me – it was more than just pain and my sanity involved. I have functioned with pains and aches so long and still had my bout with mental stress here and there. True – on a bad day nothing made me feel better mentally than fresh French fries and ketchup – it was comforting. You get used to chronic neck aches and joint pain like it was just another day. It was a liberating wakeup call to literally wake up and not feel extreme pain, or aches or fatigue from sleeping badly. For me, eliminating Nightshades helped with my inflammation a lot. I have MRIs showing the difference from when I ate these plant family members versus after 3 years of not consuming them. I would not trade that feeling for perceived comfort food ever again. I found new comfort foods that make me feel even better than that in other food families.

8 NUTS & SEEDS

Nuts and Seeds are two of the key food families that made up early man's diet. Over time as humans cultivated fire and became more hunters than gatherers, the nuts and seed were consumed less. In times where animal protein could not be found, we would revert back to the standby protein that got us through and nourished us.

Over the evolution our own species, individuals have become more allergic and sensitive to nuts and seeds. Knowing which ones are similar can significantly help during an allergic episode (IgE immune response). There are so many wonderful benefits to nuts and seeds as well as some cautions, so let's investigate further.

> **Example** : *I was never allergic to nuts as a young child. I used to eat walnuts, almonds and pistachios with ease. I was never fond of other nuts as they would taste weird to me, so I never paid it any mind. Then I got stung by a yellow jacket at the pool at my apartment complex when I was 13 and had a significantly bad reaction; my hands and feet swelled for over a week. After that, I was the poster child for allergy elimination diet, of which practically everything I ate gave me hives or made my swelling worse. This restricted and reduced diet went on for 6 months and I slowly brought foods back into my diet – the ones that did not come back were shellfish/crustaceans and nuts. I considered myself lucky that those two areas were all that was left and would always be packing antihistamine just to be sure.*

In my late 20s, I was eating crab and lobster again; however nuts still eluded my diet. A sliver of an almond got into a salad accidentally and when my throat started to itch and swell, it was a surprise indeed. I had myself re-checked with a RAST test (IgE) after the birth of my first son to find out – neither allergy showed up. I was still leery to that thought of eating those things and figured better safe than sorry and avoid it. A few months later, I started getting the same reaction with shrimp and lobster again, and so I gathered there must be a bigger issue. Another accidental nut ingestion with itchy scalp, throat and wheezing – now I was sure that the test had to have been wrong or just not evaluating the correct immune response. To this day, I am back to avoiding nuts at all costs, crustaceans and especially those pesky yellow jackets which I believe triggered this mess in the first place ☺

However, the most telling thing during my first detoxification cleanse and elimination diet over 3 years ago was my food family discovery where nuts are concerned. I cannot have almonds – ok; what family are almonds in? I had never asked that question before; almonds are in the Prune subfamily of ROSE. What other plants are in that family – and do they possess similar chemistry? I had been eating prunes and peaches a lot and still felt odd and bloated afterwards – I was hoping the extra fiber would help and it did not. It was the amygdalins in the stone fruits similar to what is found with almond that was still hurting my health. Elimination of those fruits for me produces a world of relief digestively. This would not be the first time or the last I would ask the food family question.

This is my story about nuts; if you have similar issues with nuts – it may not be the same as mine – however just ask the question and investigate further.

NUTS

Nuts are considered a dry one-seeded fruit part of a plant. They are similar to seeds as they possess the reproductive material to produce a new plant. Nature has provided a mechanism to protect that future plant – shells and husks.

The following families discussed in this chapter may have additional fruit or vegetable members as well. Those non-nut plant members will be discussed in their appropriate sections.

Cashew -- *Family Anacardiaceae* – consists of cashews, pistachios, and mango fruit. It is unusual to think cashews and pistachios were in the same family, much less mangoes. Two unique nuts – one with shell, one without and both chock full of healthy goodness.

High in Vitamins – Pistachios are high in Vitamin E (Alpha Tocopherol), Thiamine, B6. Cashews have those vitamins as well, just not as high a concentration.

High in Minerals – Cashew have very high Copper and strong Magnesium, Manganese, and Zinc; Pistachios have strong Copper, Manganese, Potassium and Phosphorus.

Amino Acids Completeness – Both nuts have a complete amino acid profile to support necessary protein consumption in your diet.

Consumption Profile	Cashews (100 g)	Pistachios (100 g)
Protein	18.2 g	20.6 g
Fat	43.8 g	44.4 g
Carbohydrates	32.7 g	28.0 g
Fiber	3.3 g	10.3 g

Key Chemical components – Pistachios have lignans; Cashews have plant sterols, stanol esters, tannins; Antibacterial elements of anacardic acid, cardol and cardanol found in the cashew nutshell liquid (a by-product of processing the cashew for consumption); Urushiol.

Reasons to consume: Both nuts are anti-inflammatory (due to monounsaturated fats) to our diets and have low glycemic load. Remember since nuts are nutrient dense, consuming them in moderation is strongly recommended. Pistachios phytoestrogens have been shown to reduce cholesterol. Cashews are considered antimicrobial, antibacterial, and anti-cytotoxic. Both nuts have shown to decrease the risk of certain cancers.

Reasons not to consume: Cashews must be well cleaned and shelled as their shell is highly toxic in order to be consumed. This nut family possesses an allergenic oil urushiol which is also a toxin found in the related plant poison ivy, sumac, etc. Also pistachios are exposed to Aflatoxin just like with peanuts due to poor harvesting practices or unsanitary processing. Cashews are metabolic inhibitors to Blood Type A and can have negative impact to Blood Type O disease sensitivities. Pistachios impair gastric functions and prevent assimilation of nutrients in A and O blood types.

છ છ છ

Palm -- *Family Arecaceae* – consists of palm oil, sago, coconut, hearts of palm and dates. Coconut is technically a fruit that is similar in makeup to nuts and when consumed can be as difficult to digest in equal quantity to nuts.

High in Vitamins – None.

High in Minerals – Manganese.

Amino Acid Completeness – Mostly complete, though insufficient amino acids for a complete protein source the diet.

Consumption Profile	Coconut (100 g)
Protein	3.3 g
Fat	33.5 g
Carbohydrates	15.2 g
Fiber	9.0 g

Key Chemical components – Medium chain triglycerides (MCTs); also contains lauric, myristic, palmitic, caprylic and oleic acids.

Reasons to consume: MCTs are beneficial to balancing the cholesterol in the body – they do not convert to trans-fats when cooking with coconut oil. Protects the liver from alcohol damage. Lauric and Caprylic acids are antibacterial, anti-viral, anti-fungal and anti-protozoal. Fruit juice and water from a green coconut is used as a remedy for poisoning and cholera. Coconut water plus rice flour combined can be used as a poultice for carbuncles, sores and ulcers.

Reasons not to consume: It is high in saturated fats - 29.7 grams of the 33.5 grams per 100 gram serving. Additionally, coconut by-products and derivatives have been known to cause contact dermatitis.

CS CS CS

Birch -- *Family Betulaceae* – consists of filberts and hazelnuts. There is very little difference between the two, as one is grown in Europe and the other is from North America. These plants are cultivated for their edible nuts. The nuts that are predominately consumed are the European species. This is not to be confused with *Witch Hazel* as it is a different plant family all together.

High in Vitamins – Vitamin E* (Alpha Tocopherol), Thiamine, B6, Folate.

High in Minerals – Copper*, Magnesium*, Manganese*, and Phosphorus.

Amino Acid Completeness – Incomplete amino acid protein structure – needs to be complemented with other protein to obtain complete nutrients.

Consumption Profile	Filberts/Hazelnuts – (100 g)
Protein	15.0 g
Fat	60.7 g
Carbohydrates	16.7 g
Fiber	9.7 g

Key Chemical components – Oleic acid, phytosterol (beta-sitosterol) and antioxidant phenolics such as catechins.

Reasons to consume: Low in cholesterol and sodium. Significant source of monounsaturated fats. These nuts are a strongly anti-inflammatory food.

Reasons not to consume: Higher in Omega-6 than Omega-3 fatty acids so one should eat in moderation. B Blood types have issues with hazelnuts/filberts due to the agglutination of proteins in the blood – essentially the protein drops out of the cells, making it difficult to carry the nutrients that would bind there.

ೞ ೞ ೞ

Chestnut -- *Family Fagaceae* – consists of beechnut, **chestnuts** and oak acorns. During the middle ages in southern Europe, the forest centric communities depended on chestnuts as their main source of carbohydrates. Access to wheat was scarce so chestnuts were milled into flour.

High in Vitamins – These nuts are the only one high in Vitamin C. There is also B and K vitamin, just not in high quantities.

High in Minerals – Manganese.

Amino Acid Completeness – Chestnuts have a complete amino acid profile to support necessary protein consumption in your diet

Consumption Profile	Chestnuts (100 g)
Protein	3.2 g
Fat	2.2 g
Carbohydrates	53.0 g
Fiber	5.1 g

Key Chemical components: Enzyme Chitinase; tannins, plastoquinones, and mucilage.

Reasons to consume: Consumption of roasted chestnuts roasted is said to support recovery of whooping cough, bronchitis and sore throat. It is also documented to facilitate blood circulation, support the kidney and stomach functions and reduce inflammation.

Reasons not to consume: The Chitinase is thought to have a cross reaction with food and latex rubber allergies – as this is the enzyme which breaks down the shells of insects to prevent them from eating the plants.

Cʒ Cʒ Cʒ

Walnut -- *Family Juglandaceae* – consists of butternut, hickory nut, walnut, and pecan. Walnuts and pecans are two of the top five hardest nuts to digest.

High in Vitamins – Pecan are high in Thiamine; both have trace Choline and Betaine.

High in Minerals – Both nuts have Copper and Manganese*; Pecans also have Flouride and Zinc.

Amino Acid Completeness – Incomplete amino acid protein structure – needs to be complemented with other protein to obtain complete nutrients.

Consumption Profile	Walnut (100 g)	Pecan (100 g)
Protein	15.2 g	10.0 g
Fat	65.2 g	78.5 g
Carbohydrates	13.7 g	15.3 g
Fiber	6.7 g	10.5 g

Key Chemical components – both nuts have large amounts Omega-6, Omega-3 fatty acids and phytosterols; Walnuts have ellagic acid is a flavonoid and caffeic acid which are antioxidants.

Reasons to consume: These nuts are called brain food because the shape of walnuts and pecans actually mimics the lobes and structure of our brains. The Doctrine of Signatures states that the fats in both of these nuts are similar in structure to the fats used in the brain and consumption of those nuts is beneficial to the brain's balance. The essential fatty acids help regulate the Serotonin levels in the brain. In their raw form, walnuts are found to have the highest total level of antioxidants, including both free antioxidants and antioxidants bound to fiber.

Reasons not to consume: Higher inflammatory effects to our diets due to high Omega-6 to Omega-3 essential fatty acid (EFA) ratios.

CB CB CB

Brazil nut -- *Family Lecythidaceae* – consists of the Brazil nut. The tree resembles a coconut in structure and produces a ball of which the actual "nut" is one of 6-8 seeds within it. The nut is named from the plant's origin in Brazil.

High in Vitamins – Vitamin E, (Alpha Tocopherol) Thiamine and has trace amounts of Choline and Betaine.

High in Minerals – Copper, Magnesium*, Manganese, Phosphorus, Selenium*, and Zinc.

Amino Acid Completeness – Incomplete amino acid protein structure – needs to be complemented with other protein to obtain complete nutrients.

Consumption Profile	Brazil Nut (100 g)
Protein	14.3 g
Fat	66.4 g
Carbohydrates	12.3 g
Fiber	7.5 g

Key Chemical components – Omega-6 essential fatty acids, very small Omega-3 in proportion to Omega-6; highest concentration of phytic acid based on dry weight.

Reasons to consume: Highest concentration of Selenium in any member of the plant family.

Reasons not to consume: High in saturated fats. This makes these nuts moderately inflammatory to our diet due to high Omega-6 content.

CB CB CB

Pine Nuts -- *Family Pinaceae* – consist of pine nuts or also called Pignoli or Pinyon nuts. These nuts are in the center of several varieties of pine cone of evergreen plants – the most commonly known one is the Stone Pine tree. This is one of the top five hardest to digest nuts.

High in Vitamins – E (Alpha Tocopherol), K; good source of Choline and Betaine.

High in Minerals – Copper, Magnesium, Manganese*, Phosphorus and Zinc.

Amino Acid Completeness – Incomplete amino acid protein structure – needs to be complemented with other protein to obtain complete nutrients.

Consumption Profile	Pine Nuts (100 g)
Protein	13.7 g
Fat	68.4 g
Carbohydrates	13.1 g
Fiber	3.7 g

Key Chemical components: Omega-6 essential fatty acids (oleic acid), very small Omega-3 in proportion to Omega-6; Pinolenic acid.

Reasons to consume: Pinolenic acid has been shown to have appetite curbing effects by releasing cholecystokinin (CCK) into the gut helping to signal the "'full" message to the brain.

Reasons not to consume: Moderately inflammatory to our diet due to high Omega-6 content; can also cause taste alteration in some folks which can last up to a week before resolving. They have allergic cross-reactivity with the *Anacardiaceae* family (see Cashew family above).

ෆ ෆ ෆ

Macadamia -- *Family Proteaceae* – consists of the macadamia nut. This nut is part of an evergreen tree, and is the number one hardest to digest nut due to its high fat content. It is also has the lowest protein value in the family of nuts.

High in Vitamins – Thiamine.

High in Minerals – Copper, Magnesium, Manganese*, and Phosphorus.

Amino Acid Completeness – Extremely incomplete: requires other supporting components for consumption to support protein needs in your diet.

Consumption Profile	Macadamia Nut (100 g)
Protein	7.8 g
Fat*	76.1 g
Carbohydrates	13.4 g
Fiber	8.0 g

Key Chemical components: Phytosterols; Also a special EFA Omega-7 Palmitoleic Acid

Reasons to consume: Strongly anti-inflammatory to your diet – high in monounsaturated fats.

Reasons not to consume: High in saturated fats due to the Omega 7 EFA. *Note for pets* – These nuts are toxic for dogs to consume and cause temporary paralysis for between 12-24 hours. Seek medical assistance for your pet if this occurs.

ᐇ   ᐇ   ᐇ

Rose/Plum --*Family Roseaceae, Sub Family Amygdaloideae, Genus Prunoideae* – consists of plum, prune, cherry, almond******, nectarine, apricot, greengage persimmon, pluot, sloe and peach.

** Only sweet almonds will be covered in this chapter. The remaining fruits will be discussed in Chapter 10, Commonly Consumed Fruits and Vegetable.

High in Vitamins – E (Alpha Tocopherol)*, Riboflavin and Choline.

High in Minerals – Calcium, Copper, Magnesium*, Manganese*, Phosphorus*, Zinc.

Amino Acid Completeness – incomplete: requires other supporting protein components to support protein needs in your diet.

Consumption Profile	Almond – 100g
Protein	21.9 g
Fat	50.6 g
Carbohydrates	19.9 g
Fiber	10.4 g

Key Chemical components – Omega-6 fatty acids; phytosterols; flavonoids – catechin, epicatchin, kaempferol and quercetin; salicylates.

Reasons to consume: Mildly anti-inflammatory to your diet; the flavonoids are antioxidant preventing oxidant induced cell destruction.

Almonds have the total flavonoid concentration of a red onion, the catechins of green tea and the quercetin of broccoli. Also supports lowering of cholesterol. Also these nuts can be used to create a "raw milk" substitute by soaking blanched almonds in water and then blending and straining.

Reasons not to consume: High in Omega-6 without any Omega-3 component. Also can be exposed like other nuts to Aflatoxin due to poor processing or mold exposure during harvesting.

SEEDS

Technically, seeds are the ripened ovules of plants and that is where the key DNA of that plant is stored. From a seed, a new plant will grow. Seeds are similar to nuts as they are high in protein. For some folks with certain digestive issues like diverticulitis, the consumption of seeds is strongly discouraged. The seeds if not properly chewed or digested, can embed themselves in the pockets of inflammation in the colon and make the symptoms worse. There is recent research from Nutrition in Clinical Practice Journal which shows that the inflammation is not impacted by the seeds at all. It is the Fiber in those seeds that is needed to help with the condition. Seeds have many significant nutrients and are beneficial in one's diet. Let's discuss each seed family more specifically.

> **In essence all nuts are seeds, however not all seeds are nuts.**

Hemp -- *Family Cannabaceae* – consists of hemp seed and hops. Hemp is used for its fibers and its seed to produce milk or be consumed as is. More recently hemp is used for industrial purposes including paper, textiles, clothing, biodegradable plastics, body products, health food and bio-fuel. hemp seeds come from the hemp plant. This is used to describe the low tetrahydrocannabinol (THC) varieties of the plant *Cannabis sativa*.

Hops are the female flowers (also called seed cones or strobiles) of a hop species, *Humulus lupulus*. They are used primarily as a flavoring and stability agent in beer, to which they impart a bitter, tangy flavor.

High in Vitamins – Vitamin E.

High in Minerals – Calcium.

Amino Acid Completeness – Hemp seed is considered complete as it contains the 21 known amino acids, including the 9 essential ones that cannot be produced by our adult bodies. One tablespoon of hemp oil contains the proper proportions to meet the human daily requirements of Essential Fatty Acids.

Consumption Profile	Hemp Seeds (100 g)
Protein	30.6 g
Fat	47.2 g
Carbohydrates	10.9 g
Fiber	6.0 g

Key Chemical components – 44% of the weight in of hemp seed is edible oils containing approximately 80% essential fatty acids: Omega-6 linoleic acid, Omega-3 alpha linolenic acid, Omega-6 gamma-linolenic acid, and stearidonic acid. Also contains two key proteins Albumin and Edestin; Edestin is second highest in concentration in hemp seed next to soy.

Reasons to consume: "Overall, Hemp`s main nutritional advantage over other seeds lies in the composition of its oil," according to Gero Leson, D.Env., an environmental scientist and consultant with extensive experience in the food and fiber uses of hemp and other renewable resources. Hemp seeds protein also has a similar cellular structure to a protein (Albumin) manufactured in human blood, making it easily digestible. The hemp nut is also rich in the vitamin E complex of tocopherols and many trace minerals; there is no other nut or seed which provides such a density of beneficial nutrients.

Reasons not to consume: The typical Western diet contains too much Linolenic Acid and not enough Alpha Linolenic Acid essential fats. According to National Institute of Health studies and reports on the subject, this has been found to be an unhealthy balance, and the addition of good essential fatty acids has proven to help with many modern ailments such as diabetes, heart disease and metabolic syndromes. Essentially everything in a balance; of all the seeds, Hemp is by far the most desirable ratio of Omega-3/Omega-6 for consumption.

ᘓ ᘓ ᘓ

Daisy -- *Family Compositae* – composed of many leaf lettuce and flowering plants of which notable for this section is the sunflower and its seeds. Another notable seed is safflower and is used for producing safflower oil.

High in Vitamins – B6, E*, Folate, and Pantothenic Acid.

High in Minerals – Copper, Magnesium, Manganese, Phosphorus, Selenium and Zinc.

Amino Acid Completeness – Average completeness – need another protein based food to yield a complete protein source.

Consumption Profile	Sunflower Seeds (100 g)
Protein* - up to 50% composition	26.8 g
Fat	3.0 g
Carbohydrates	25.8 g
Fiber	4.4 g

* Notably high in content

Key Chemical components – Unsaturated fatty acids – higher Omega-6 vs Omega-3 (arachidic acid, eicosenic acid, linolenic acid, margaric acid, myristic acid, oleic acid, palmitic acid, palmitoleic acid, phenolic acid, stearic acid), phytosterols (plant sterols/stanol esters), lignans.

Reasons to consume: Alleviates constipation, assists healing of cuts and bruises, anti-dysentery, tonic to bodily fluids, lowers risk of hormone dependant cancers, decreases total and LDL cholesterol levels, low in cholesterol and sodium.

Reasons not to consume: For those folks who are sensitive to flowers in the Daisy family, consumption of the seed may increase allergic reaction; may promote eruptions of measles rash for those who are susceptible; strongly inflammatory food and contains trans-fats.

Ⅽⅾ　Ⅽⅾ　Ⅽⅾ

Gourd -- *Family Cucurbitaceae* – The seeds of a pumpkin, also called Pepitas, are part of the Gourd family. The pumpkin seed has a fibrous shell around it and inside is the heart of the nutrients. That green nutrient has been called Pepitas in comparison to the unshelled seed (white-yellow in color).

High in Vitamins – E (Gamma Tocopherol), and K.

High in Minerals – Copper, Iron*, Magnesium*, Manganese*, Phosphorus* and Zinc.

Amino Acids completeness – Complete – all high levels of amino acids in a strong protein structure.

Consumption Profile	Pumpkin Seeds 1 cup (138 g)
Protein* - over 50% composition	33.9 g
Fat*	63.3 g
Carbohydrates	24.6 g
Fiber	5.4 g

* Notably high in content

Key Chemical components – Unsaturated fatty acids with higher Omega-6 vs Omega-3 (linolenic acid, oleic acid, palmitic acid, stearic acid).

Reasons to consume: Diuretic effect and reduce hypertrophy of prostate, anthelmintic (cucubitine); low in cholesterol and sodium.

Reasons not to consume: High in fat, and as with all seeds, should be eaten in moderation; moderately inflammatory food.

⅓ ⅓ ⅓

Flax -- *Family Linaceae* – Consists of flaxseed. Flaxseed is also known as linseed. This is a classified as powerful food, due to its high concentration of essential fatty acids that our body needs to facilitate our bodily processes. Flax used to be one of those "new-age" health nut kind of foods; now it is mainstream and found in commercial products more and more.

High in Vitamins – Thiamine* and B6.

High in Minerals – Copper*, Magnesium*, Manganese*, Phosphorus* Selenium and Zinc.

Amino Acids Completeness – Slightly incomplete – need another protein source food to yield a complete protein profile.

Consumption Profile	Flaxseed 1 cup (168 g)
Protein	30.7 g
Fat*	70.8 g
Carbohydrates	48.5 g
Fiber	45.9 g

Key Chemical components – Highest concentration of Omega-3 EFA found in any plant.

Reasons to consume: Flax is the most anti-inflammatory seed to consume. Flax also has antibacterial, anticancer, and anti-viral properties. Great to substitute for eggs in baking, due to the natural mucilage produced when soaking the seeds.

Reasons not to consume: This seed has been shown to be genetically modified in its mass production. Please make sure to source organically to ensure no potential issues. Remember this is a fragile seed oil and needs to be refrigerated to ensure it does not spoil; can last up to 6 months in refrigerator or freezer.

℃ ℃ ℃

Mint -- Family Lamiaceae – Consists of chia seeds. It is one of the flowering members of this family. Chia is grown for its seed to be used similar to flaxseed in drinks and food products. Yes it is the same plant in the CHIA PETS, except that the plant has not flowered.

High in Vitamins – None.

High in Minerals – Calcium, Manganese and Phosphorus.

Amino Acid Completeness – Chia has a complete amino acid protein structure – nothing needs to be added to obtain complete nutrients.

Consumption Profile	Chia Seed 1 ounce (28 g)
Protein	4.4 g
Fat	8.6 g
Carbohydrates	12.3 g
Fiber	10.6 g

Key Chemical components – Omega -3 and Omega-6 EFA.

Reasons to consume: Chia is mildly anti-inflammatory to our health. Great to substitute for eggs in baking, due to the natural mucilage produced when soaking the seeds.

Reasons not to consume: No particular reason other than similar problems with sesame or flaxseed. Even with the mucilaginous coating, chia seeds may get embedded in inflamed tissue of the colon.

ᘓ ᘓ ᘓ

Sesame -- *Family Pedaliaceae* – Consists of sesame seed. Don't let the size fool you on how beneficial this seed is; Size does not matter here!

High in Vitamins – Thiamine, B6.

High in Minerals – Calcium*, Copper*, Iron*, Magnesium*, Manganese*, Phosphorus, and Zinc.

Amino Acids completeness: Low on the incomplete amino acid protein structure – needs to be complemented with other protein to obtain complete nutrients.

Consumption Profile	Sesame Seeds 1 cup (144 g)
Protein	25.5 gram
Fat*	71.5 gram
Carbohydrates	33.8 gram
Fiber	17.0 gram

* Notably high in content

Key Chemical components – Unsaturated fatty acids and Sesamin, a phytoestrogen.

Reasons to consume: Low in cholesterol and sodium. Sesame seeds contain a special phytoestrogen called Sesamin. This may help Vitamin E curb the production of inflammatory alkaloids called Eicosanoids. Eicosanoids are produced when there is too much Omega-6 and not enough Omega-3s in the diet. As a result, the immune functions can be impaired.

Reasons not to consume: This is one of the seeds that are considered to be highly allergic/sensitive to some folks. It is also found to be slightly inflammatory due to the overwhelming concentration of Omega-6 versus Omega-3 fatty acids. The high oil content makes this susceptible to spoilage quickly – refrigeration can extend life up to 6 months, freezing up to a year; don't forget to smell them before consuming.

Food Combination – NUTS & SEEDS

As nutrient dense foods, nuts and seed take longer to digest compared to other grasses and legumes. Nuts have key phenolic acids and phytic acid in them which are antioxidant and anti-carcinogenic. Their chemical composition is more complex as well – average of 45% fats, 25% proteins, 20% carbohydrates and less than 10% water. Protein and fats are most difficult to break down and digest properly. Nuts and seeds possess oils which are the basis of the high fat percentage and without modern processing equipment, mass consumption would not be possible.

Nuts and seeds are produced with shells covering them, and those shells for the most part are not digestible, hence signaling – eat with care and not so many. Mother Nature planned for nuts and seeds to be eaten one at a time, not en-masse. Today, thousands of nuts or seeds are found in a jar of their respective butters or in a carton of nut and seed milks. These processed products are forms of concentrated oil, protein and carbohydrate which can still be difficult to digest. However when presented with a dairy free need – nut and seed milks are the excellent substitutes compared to rice, oat or soy. Those nuts that are extremely high in fats will be the hardest to digest – top five are macadamia, pine, Brazil, pecan and walnut.

The best form to consume nuts and seeds is fresh out of shell (raw or roasted) to ensure there has been no oxidation from heat light and air. Once nuts are shelled, their protective armor is gone and their delicate oils are subject to rancidity. Rancid oils and fats when consumed are a source of free radicals in the body. If you smell the tell tale sour odor, its best to discard the nuts immediately. Free radicals decompose into peroxides and aldehydes, which are known carcinogens which are harmful to our health.

It is strongly suggested to refrigerate nuts and seeds to prolong their usability without compromising their fragile oil structures. For example, flaxseed needs to be refrigerated whether it is ground or whole. The sour smell of rancid oil in nuts and seeds is easy to discern. If you smell that or it has that off smell, better to discard.

When nuts are prominent in a full sized meal, it can take *longer* (between 2 and 3 hours) for the stomach to empty due to the extra digestion processing.

Did you know - Peanuts are not NUTS, they are LEGUMES. It is easy to confuse the point as there are so many nut allergies. Nut allergies are for specific tree based nuts, ones which have pollen impacts from the pollination of the trees in the Summer and Fall. Please refer to the Legume section for more information on peanuts and their allergies and sensitivities.

The following plants and/or animals are evaluated to combine with nuts & seeds:

Excellent – Lettuce Family, dried Fruits, non-starchy vegetables
Good – Animal and Dairy Families
Poor – Grass Family, Legume Family, other starches, Fungi

Pollen interactions when consuming Nuts and Seeds

Can inhaling specific pollens exacerbate allergic or sensitive reaction to foods consumed? Additionally, can having a specific condition increase the sensitivity or reactions to food? Dr. Jacqueline Krohn and other physicians have documented examples of these occurrences.

Pollen/Condition	*Food Family/Members*
Dust and Viral Infections	*All Nuts & Seeds*

Blood Type Impacts

Dr. Peter D'Adamo has documented reactions of foods to health, based on blood type in *Eat Right for your Type*. If you follow the specifics below for A or B blood types and still have issues, you may be a mixed blood type (part A or B and part O). Please refer to the Let's Get Started section to review for more information about mixed blood types. It would be best to evaluate both blood types' food specifics and see where your reactions lie.

Nuts & Seeds to Avoid by Blood Type			
O	A	B	AB
Brazil Nut	Brazil Nut	Cashew/Cashew Butter	Filberts (Hazelnuts)
Cashew/Cashew Butter	Cashew/Cashew Butter	Filberts (Hazelnuts)	Poppy Seed
Litchi	Pistachio	Pine Nut	Pumpkin Seed
Pistachio		Pistachio	Sesame Butter/ Tahini/ Sesame Seed
Poppy Seed		Poppy Seed	Sunflower Seed/Butter
Sunflower Seed/Butter		Pumpkin Seed	
		Sesame Butter/ Tahini/ Sesame Seed	
		Sunflower Seed/Butter	

Nuts & Seeds that are Beneficial by Blood Type			
O	A	B	AB
Almond/Almond Butter	Flax Seed	Walnuts	Chestnut
Flax Seed	Pumpkin Seed		Walnuts
Pumpkin Seed	Walnuts		
Walnuts			

All other nuts not listed in tables have a neutral impact by blood types.

> *In general, Blood Type **B** is the most susceptible to Nut & Seed allergies and intolerances. Walnuts are the only member of the Nut & Seed families which can be consumed by Blood Type B, and is beneficial for all blood types as well.*

General Foodergies™ Issues

Nuts in general are not inter-related to each other at all, yet most people who are allergic to one, tend to be allergic to all. It can be inferred that because of how they are created – in shells – that certain chemical components are present to prevent rotting or spoiling, enduring long periods of time before germination. It is those potentially common chemicals that are 'shared' among the nut family members. Common allergic symptoms of nuts can be excess mucus, respiratory issues like asthma, anaphylactic shock, and severe headaches like migraines or digestive issues. My theory goes back to the similar pollens during the plant's reproductive process – and for those who have pollen allergies or sensitivities as well as nut, that it is the presence of pollen interacting with the proteins which make it one of those Foodergies™. This could also be said for the seeds as well.

Dr. Jonathan Brostoff documents the relationship between specific tree pollens and nuts / seeds as follows:

- Birch Pollen – hazelnut, walnut, Rose family (almonds)
- Mugwort Pollen – Rose family (almonds)
- Ragweed – sunflower seeds, coconut
- Pine – pine nuts
- Hazel – hazelnuts

9 FUNGI

The Fungi are an interesting food family to investigate. They are not truly "alive" in the same context as plants or animal as they function through anaerobic means – without air. They reproduce through spreading their spores (similar to seeds) through the air and flourish on the rotting of wood or mulch, in the damp and dark.

For some, this does not sound appetizing in the least. For others, it is a deeply connected sharing in the biological circle of life; nutrients broken down, feeding into to other creatures, and returning benefits back into the soil and earth. Regardless of the perspective, the Fungi play a meaningful role in the foods we eat and in return our bodies may or may not respond in favorable kind.

Members of the family: Mushrooms (shiitake, maitake, enoki, straw, white, portabello, crimini, black trumpet, oyster/abalone, to name a few), brewer's yeast and baker's yeast, (beneficial bacterias in culturing) and probiotics

Commonly used ways these members are found and consumed: Farmed and wild cultivated Mushrooms; Yeast produces beers, lager, and breads; Beneficial bacteria cultured or fermented products like Kefir, yogurt, and sauerkraut; Probiotic supplements, some exclusively sourced with Yeast used to treat Candida overgrowth and intestinal distress - e.g. FloraStor is the commercial name for a strain similar to the baker's/brewer's yeast named *Saccharomyces boulardii*.

High in Vitamins –

Mushrooms – Riboflavin, Niacin, Folate, Vitamin D (In Shiitake Mushrooms).

Brewer's / Baker's Yeast – B-Vitamin Complex.

Probiotics – None.

High in Minerals –

Mushrooms – Selenium, Potassium. Lithium.

Brewer's / Baker's Yeast – Brewer's Yeast Chromium and Selenium; except for Baker's Yeast – Selenium only.

Probiotics – None.

> ***NOTE****: Some folks are under the assumption that Brewer's Yeast / Baker's Yeast / Nutritional Yeast have **natural** B12. **It does not**. The B12 is synthesized outside of the Yeast budding process and supplemented.*

Amino Acids Completeness – Fungi (Mushrooms) have an incomplete amino acid profile; other additional proteins need to be consumed to support necessary amino acid requirements in your diet. Baker's and Brewer's yeast however have full amino acid profile on their own.

Consumption Profile	Portabello Mushroom 1 cup diced (86 g)	Straw Mushroom 1 cup, strained (182 g)	Domestic White Mushroom– 1 cup diced (70 g)
Protein	2.2 g	7.0 g	2.2 g
Fat	0.2 g	1.2 g	0.2 g
Carbohydrates	4.4 g	8.4 g	2.3 g
Fiber	1.3 g	4.6 g	0.7 g

Consumption Profile	Enoki Mushroom 1 medium (3 g)	Shiitake Mushroom 1 dried piece (3 g)	Maitake Mushroom– 1 cup diced (70 g)
Protein	0.1 g	0.3 g	1.4 g
Fat	0.0 g	0.0 g	0.1 g
Carbohydrates	0.2 g	2.6 g	4.8 g
Fiber	0.1 g	0.4 g	1.9 g

Consumption Profile	Crimini Mushroom 1 piece (20 g)	Abalone-Oyster Mushroom 1 large (14.8 g)	Black Trumpet Mushroom– (100 g)
Protein	0.5 g	4.9 g	9.0 g
Fat	0.0 g	0.6 g	0.0 g
Carbohydrates	0.8 g	9.6 g	75.0 g
Fiber	0.1 g	3.4 g	12.0 g

Consumption Profile	Brewer's-Baker's Yeast 1 tbsp (8 g)
Protein	4.6 g
Fat*	0.6 g
Carbohydrates	4.6 g
Fiber	2.5 g

Key Chemical components – Members of the Fungi family all have Omega-3 & 6, Choline and Betaine.

Reasons to consume:

Mushrooms – They have Omega-3 and 6 to support our EFA needs; Lithium for neurological balance. Additionally mushrooms have anti-viral and immune system enhancing properties. Mushrooms have very high concentrations of Ergothioneine. Ergothioneine is considered an antioxidant and anti-inflammatory. This powerful compound is released during the cooking process. This gives mushrooms an antioxidant level greater than green pepper and zucchini. Shiitake mushrooms have two key compounds called Lenthionin and Eritadenine. Lenthionin prevents platelets from clumping and may help reduce the chance for thrombosis. Eritadenine is being investigated to lower blood cholesterol levels acting as a stimulant or suppressor in our tissues.

When cut mushrooms look like our ears and with the Vitamin D in them support the bones in our body as well as our ears to maintain our hearing. It appears that mushrooms respond like we do in the synthesis of D3. Mushrooms' levels of Vitamin D can be enhanced by exposing them to Ultraviolet light. The D2 came from a different form of D than we produce as part of the Vitamin D synthesis process. The ergosterol is converted to D2. This is similar to humans where D3 is synthesized by exposure to sun light.

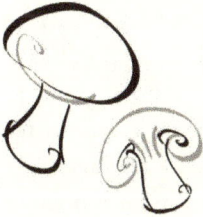

Brewer's / Baker's Yeast – Complete amino acid source and beneficial to supporting digestion, in moderation.

Probiotics – the group of bacteria that are cultivated to support the balancing of the intestinal flora is considered strongly beneficial. The majority of the population complains of one sort of lower digestive upset or discomfort. The addition of probiotics can help alleviate some of those symptoms. Additionally, cultured foods contain specific kinds of bacteria / fungi which help keep the sensitive colon flora balance in check. Also probiotics help keep the colon in balance when one is taking antibiotics for infections. Ccurrent evidence supports the efforts of probiotics in balancing the gut microbes; preventing invasion of toxins and unfriendly microbes in the gut; alleviating diarrhea, Irritable Bowel Syndrome, lactose intolerance, and *Helicobacter pylori* infection; balancing the immune function; and possibly supporting prevention of colon cancer.

Reasons not to consume:

Mushrooms - If one has allergies to mold, consuming members of this family may make your allergies worse; some mushroom species are actually subject to mold contamination (Shiitake and black trumpets, for example) and it is best to look for organic options. Straw and domestic white mushrooms have lectins which may cause digestive issues. Also raw mushrooms contain a compound called Agaritine which can be carcinogenic in large quantities. It is present in raw mushrooms but is destroyed when cooked.

Brewer's / Baker's Yeast & Probiotics – If you have a compromised colon and have no idea what is causing it, taking probiotics may upset the balance even more depending on what is deficient. Most Candida (opportunistic pathogenic yeast) infestations have been known to respond well to *Saccharomyces boulardii*; other folks may just be irregular in their bowels for other reasons. It is advisable to choose a particular species or strain of a probiotic for a health-maintenance or need. Not all multi strain probiotics formulas have the same properties and activities. One needs to be aware that animal studies have shown there is an upper safe limit of probiotic consumption.

Food Combination – FUNGI

The best form to consume Fungi is fresh or cooked. When Fungi are prominent in a full sized meal, it can take between 1 - 2 hours for the stomach to process.

The following plants and/or animals are evaluated to combine with Fungi:

Excellent – Lettuce family, dried Fruits, non-starchy vegetables
Good – Animal and Dairy Families, (except for beef with yeast)
Poor – Grass Family, Legume Family, nuts & seeds, other starches, beef with yeast

Pollen interactions when consuming Fungi

Can inhaling specific pollens exacerbate allergic or sensitive reaction to foods consumed? Additionally, can having a specific condition increase the sensitivity or reactions to food? Dr. Jacqueline Krohn and other physicians have documented examples of these occurrences.

Pollen/Condition	Food Family/Members
Cedar Pollen, Juniper Pollen and Candida Overgrowth	Fungi

Blood Type Impacts

Dr. Peter D'Adamo has documented reactions of foods to health based on blood type in **Eat Right for your Type**. If you follow the specifics below for A or B blood types and still have issues, you may be a mixed blood type (part A or B and part O). Please refer to the Let's Get Started section to review for more information about mixed blood types. It would be best to evaluate both blood types' food specifics and see where your reactions lie.

Fungi to Avoid by Blood Type			
O	A	B	AB
Shiitake	Shiitake		Shiitake
Domestic White	Domestic White		Abalone-Oyster
	Maitake		Maitake
			Black Trumpet

Fungi that are Beneficial by Blood Type			
O	A	B	AB
	Domestic White	Shiitake	

All other Fungi not listed in tables have a neutral impact by blood types.

Diabetes Supporting and Blood Types
- Black trumpet, enoki, oyster, portabello – B and AB
- Straw, shiitake – B
- Maitake – All
- White mushroom, brewer's yeast– A, B, and AB
- Baker's yeast - AB

Cancer Preventative and Blood Types
- Maitake, shiitake - A
- White mushrooms – All

General Foodergies™ Issues

Fungi have their nutritional place in the sun and a place of reverence for medicinal purposes. As a general food item for consumption in lieu of meat or other food families – it is a toss up on whether it may be worth the risk. Not every one reacts well to molds, and the mushrooms just happen to be a different manifestation of that group.

10 COMMONLY CONSUMED
FRUIT & VEGETABLES

This is the largest chapter by far of this book. Due to the large number of food families, the most commonly consumed fruits and vegetables will be singled out for consumption profiles – carbohydrates, fats, protein and fiber. Each plant family as a whole will be discussed with its benefits and potential challenges to supporting one's health.

Kiwi -- *Family Actinidiacea*: Kiwi is also known as Chinese Gooseberry. These unique fruits originated in China. They were renamed to kiwi in the early 1960's after the Kiwi bird from New Zealand as the fruit mimicked the bird's fuzzy coat.

High in Vitamins – Vitamin C and K, Choline

High in Minerals – Potassium

Amino Acids Completeness – Kiwi has an incomplete amino acid profile; other additional proteins need to be consumed to support necessary amino acid requirements in your diet.

Consumption Profile	Kiwi 1 cup raw (177 g)
Protein	2.0 g
Fat	0.9 g
Carbohydrates	25.9 g
Fiber	5.3 g

Key Chemical components – Malic Acid, Citric Acid, Salicylic Acid, Oxalates; Hydroxycinnamic acids (Antioxidant).

Reasons to consume: The antioxidant properties of kiwi have been shown to remediate asthma symptoms, and inhibiting formation of carcinogens in the body. Additionally, kiwi has anti-viral properties.

Reasons not to consume: Kiwi possesses oxalates. Foods with oxalates exacerbate gout and other rheumatic conditions. Additionally, this fruit is one of those which can trigger Oral Allergy Syndrome. Also, this fruit can trigger the Latex-Fruit Allergy symptoms as well. Cooking this fruit breaks down the enzymes which are the catalyst in the allergic response.

သ သ သ

Goosefoot/Spinach -- *Family Amaranthaceae:* Plants like spinach, beet, sugar beet, chard, amaranth and quinoa are in this family. In this section we will be talking about spinach, beet and chard. Amaranth and quinoa are discussed in Chapter 4.

High in Vitamins – Vitamin K, E, C, A, Niacin, Folate, Choline, Betaine.

High in Minerals – Calcium, Potassium, Magnesium.

Amino Acids Completeness – Spinach has a complete protein profile. Beets and Chard have an incomplete amino acid profile; other additional proteins need to be consumed to support necessary amino acid requirements in your diet.

Consumption Profile	Spinach 1 cup raw (30 g)	Beets 1 cup raw (136 g)	Swiss Chard 1 cup raw (36 g)
Protein	0.9 g	2.2 g	0.6 g
Fat	0.1 g	0.2 g	0.1 g
Carbohydrates	1.1 g	13.0 g	1.3 g
Fiber	0.7 g	3.8 g	0.6 g

Key Chemical components – Lithium is found in the greens of beets and in chard. *Solanine* is found in sugar beets. Omega-3 & 6 is present in all of these plant members. Trimethyglycine (the original discovery of Betaine) is in its highest concentration in this family of plants; quinoa is the highest, then spinach.

Reasons to consume: Members of this family have strong antioxidant properties. Additionally, beets are anti-bacterial and chard is anticoagulant. This plant family is one of the most versatile in health benefits from fighting cancer to preventing macular degeneration. These plants are power foods.

Reasons not to consume: Beets are being genetically modified to help support the needs of sugar in commercial processing. Also the presence of solanine in this plant means it needs to be watched and evaluated for rheumatologic sensitivities.

CS CS CS

Amaryllis -- *Family Amaryllidaceae*: This food family has more than just nutritional significance. Some of these plants are used in Homeopathy to help relieve allergy symptoms of runny nose, watery eyes and congestion. Who could that be? Onion – that's who! Additionally its family member's garlic and leek have their benefits too.

High in Vitamins – Vitamin C and Choline in all three. Onion has high Folate too.

High in Minerals – Leeks are high in Manganese.

Amino Acids Completeness – Amaryllis family members have an incomplete amino acid profile; other additional proteins need to be consumed to support necessary amino acid requirements in your diet.

Consumption Profile	Onion 1 cup raw (160 g)	Garlic 3 cloves raw (9 g)	Leek 1 cup raw (89 g)
Protein	1.8 g	0.6 g	1.3 g
Fat	0.2 g	0.0 g	0.3 g
Carbohydrates	14.9 g	3.0 g	12.6 g
Fiber	2.7 g	0.2 g	1.6 g

Key Chemical components – Omega-3 & 6 and phytonutrients – allicin and allyl sulfate (organosulfurs); Quercetin.

Reasons to consume: Members of this family are anti-inflammatory foods. The possess many benefits – antibiotic, anti-viral, anticoagulant, anticancer, antioxidant, antibacterial. Garlic is used as a decongestant, expectorant and relieves intestinal gas. Onion is promoted to have sedative,

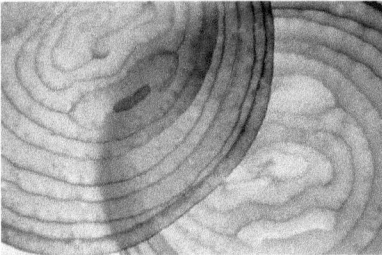

and analgesic activities. Ever notice when you slice an onion what is really looks like? The structure of an onion sliced parallel to the root shows it look like a cell. The onion helps to clear waste from our bodied; especially when they facilitate tears which bathe and clear the surface layers of our eyes.

Reasons not to consume: The organosulfur components can cause heartburn and upset stomach for those who are sulfur sensitive.

ෆ ෆ ෆ

Cashew -- *Family Anacardiaceae*: The Mango is the only fruit in this otherwise nut and shrub based family. *Cashews/pistachios are in Chapter 8.*

High in Vitamins – Vitamin C, A, E and Choline.

High in Minerals – None.

Amino Acids Completeness – Mango has an incomplete amino acid profile; other additional proteins need to be consumed to support necessary amino acid requirements in your diet.

Consumption Profile	Mango 1 cup raw sliced (165 g)
Protein	0.8 g
Fat	0.4 g
Carbohydrates	28.1 g
Fiber	3.0 g

Key Chemical components – Omega-3 & 6 with a 3:1 ratio. Phytonutrients – Lutein, mangiferin, phenolic acids – hydroxycinnamic acids and bioflavonoids – kaempferol and quercetin.

Reasons to consume: Strong antioxidant properties, which have demonstrated prevention of prostate and skin cancers.

Reasons not to consume: Can cause dermatitis from the contact of the family toxin, Urushiol. This toxin is native to this family of plants and is the same one which coats the outside of cashews. Additionally, the toxin can be the trigger for Latex-Fruit allergy and Oral Allergy Syndrome.

C3 C3 C3

Palm -- *Family Arecaceae.* Dates are not the only "fruit" from this family. Coconut is technically a fruit. However due to the very high fat content and digestive patterns, it is found with the Nuts and Seeds in Chapter 8.

High in Vitamins – None.

High in Minerals – None.

Amino Acids Completeness – Dates have an incomplete amino acid profile; other additional proteins need to be consumed to support necessary amino acid requirements in your diet.

Consumption Profile	Dates raw mature (100 g)
Protein	1.8 g
Fat	0.2 g
Carbohydrates	75.0 g
Fiber	6.7 g

Key Chemical components – antioxidants (Lutein & zeaxanthin), anthocyanins, caretenoids, tannins and phenolics

Reasons to consume: High fiber and excellent for glycemic restoration. Also this is an alkaline food with a good balance of protein and sugars. Additionally, this member possesses Salicylate activity which is beneficial for the skin.

Reasons not to consume: This is a low allergenic food. There can be a rare allergic cross reaction with Birch pollen sensitivity. Also those who are sensitive to Salicylates should avoid/reduce exposure to this food family member.

CB CB CB

Asparagus -- *Family Asparagaceae*. Asparagus is considered the "royal vegetable" as it was only served to the aristocracy. These plants are only available for a limited period of time each year due to the growing conditions necessary to produce an edible crop.

High in Vitamins – Vitamin K, A, Folate, and Choline.

High in Minerals – Iron, Copper, Lithium.

Amino Acids Completeness – Asparagus has an incomplete amino acid profile; additional other proteins need to be consumed to support necessary amino acid requirements in your diet.

Consumption Profile	Asparagus 1 cup raw (134 g)
Protein	2.9 g
Fat	0.2 g
Carbohydrates	5.3 g
Fiber	2.8 g

Key Chemical components – Bioflavonoids, key amino acid asparagine, saponins, Rutin, Asparagusic acid (a native sulfur compound), and oxalates.

Reasons to consume: Anti-inflammatory food with antioxidant and anticancer properties. Additionally this food family is known for its diuretic and laxative activity.

Reasons not to consume: The presence of oxalates requires that this food family/member be consumed with restriction as so not to exacerbate gout or rheumatic/kidney conditions. Also if there is sulfur sensitivity, it may be wise to monitor reactions and reduce consumption based on the native sulfur compound.

03 03 03

Cruciferous Greens or Mustard -- *Family Brassicaceae*. This food family is one of the most talked about today in the nutritional landscape. The most commonly consumed members are organized by species as follows:

- Arugula
- Brassica Species
  - o Oleracea groups
    - Cauliflower
    - Kale
    - Cabbage
    - Broccoli
  - o Turnip
- Radish
- Mustard Greens
- Maca Root

High in Vitamins – Vitamin K, C and Choline in all members; Kale and Mustard Greens have Vitamin A and E as well.

High in Minerals – Calcium, Lithium, Potassium.

Amino Acids Completeness – Brassicas have an incomplete amino acid profile; other additional proteins need to be consumed to support necessary amino acid requirements in your diet.

Consumption Profile	Arugula raw (100 g)	Mustard Greens ½ cup raw chopped (56 g)	Turnip 1 cup cubed raw (130 g)
Protein	2.8 g	1.5 g	1.2 g
Fat	0.7 g	0.1 g	0.1
Carbohydrates	3.7 g	2.7 g	8.4 g
Fiber	1.6 g	1.8 g	2.3 g

Consumption Profile	Cabbage 1 cup chopped raw (89 g)	Cauliflower 1 cup raw (100g)	Broccoli 1 cup raw (91 g)
Protein	1.1 g	2.0 g	2.6 g
Fat	0.1 g	0.1 g	0.3 g

Carbohydrates	5.2 g	5.3 g	6.0 g
Fiber	2.2 g	2.5 g	2.4 g

Consumption Profile	Kale 1 cup chopped raw (67 g)	Maca Root dried 1 tsp (10 g)	Radish 1 cup chopped raw (116 g)
Protein	2.2 g	1.4 g	0.8 g
Fat	0.5 g	0.2 g	0.1 g
Carbohydrates	6.7 g	7.5 g	4.0 g
Fiber	1.3 g	0.8 g	1.9 g

Key Chemical components – Indole-3-Carbinol; Even to High ratios of Omega-3 to Omega-6 in this family; Quercetin; Sulforophanes, Nicotine (in Cauliflower); phytonutrients; proanthocyanins.

Reasons to consume: This food family is by far the "powerhouse" of foods. The members of this family have antibacterial, antioxidant, anticancer, and anti-viral properties. They are all alkaline and beneficial to our bodies. These members also have other interesting uses. For example, Maca root is reported to be used as an immunostimulant similar to Ginseng. It has been used in Peru for anemia, tuberculosis, female reproductive system issues and to enhance memory. Additionally, the high sulfur members of this family are used as decongestants and expectorants besides being antibacterial.

Reasons not to consume: The natural sulforaphanes have similar issues with digestive upset and irritation as the *Amaryllidaceae* family. Also, large quantities of Maca root can cause intestinal gas.

ය ය ය

Pineapple -- *Family Bromeliaceae:* Pineapple is the only edible fruit of this plant family.

High in Vitamins – Vitamin C and Choline.

High in Minerals – Manganese.

Amino Acids Completeness – Pineapples have an incomplete amino acid profile; other additional proteins need to be consumed to support necessary amino acid requirements in your diet.

Consumption Profile	Pineapple 1 cup chunks raw (165 g)
Protein	0.9 g
Fat	0.2 g
Carbohydrates	21.6 g
Fiber	2.3 g

Key Chemical components – Bromelain, an important digestive enzyme; Phytosterols; flavonoids (antioxidants); Omega-3 & 6 with a close 1:1 ratio with Omega-6 slightly higher; Salicylates.

Reasons to consume: Strong digestive support (for gas, slow processing and heartburn) from the Bromelain; also acts as a diuretic, appetite suppressant, anti-inflammatory, anti-viral, antibacterial and anti-parasitic food.

Reasons not to consume: Acidic food to be consumed in moderation. Salicylate activity requires monitoring and reduction if having allergic / sensitivity reaction.

ଔ   ଔ   ଔ

Pawpaw -- *Family Caricaceae*. Papaya – a nutrient packed tropical fruit that is used in its various forms of ripeness.

High in Vitamins – Vitamin C.

High in Minerals – Potassium.

Amino Acids Completeness – Papaya has an incomplete amino acid profile; other additional proteins need to be consumed to support necessary amino acid requirements in your diet.

Consumption Profile	Papaya 1 cup cubed (140 g)
Protein	0.9 g
Fat	0.2 g
Carbohydrates	13.7 g
Fiber	2.5 g

Key Chemical components – Papain, a key digestive enzyme 3:1 ratio of Omega-3 to Omega-6 essential fatty acids; Carpaine, caracin – alkaloids.

Reasons to consume: This member has antibacterial and anticancer properties. Papaya – an alkaline food - is known for its supportive intestinal and digestive properties – from relieving diarrhea to removing intestinal parasites. It is also good for female hormonal issues as well. Additionally papaya is a great skin tonic providing support for the health of our skin.

Reasons not to consume: This plant has been known to show a cross reaction for Latex-Fruit Allergy. This can result in dermatitis and/or respiratory issues.

C3 C3 C3

Morning Glory -- *Family Convolvulaceae:* Sweet potato is a plant which is always confused with an unrelated family member, the yam. Each plant produces a tuber like root to consume, however these plants could not be more different. In the United States we use the term interchangeably however that does a disservice to educating the public. The "yams" we know are really sweet potatoes in species.

High in Vitamins – Vitamin A.

High in Minerals – Potassium.

Amino Acids Completeness – Sweet Potato have an incomplete amino acid profile; other additional proteins need to be consumed to support necessary amino acid requirements in your diet.

Consumption Profile	Sweet Potato 1 cup cubed (133 g)
Protein	2.1 g
Fat	0.1 g
Carbohydrates	26.8 g
Fiber	4.0 g

Key Chemical components – Omega-3 to 6 with high in Omega-6; Beta carotene (antioxidant) and other carotenoids; Caffeic acid; anthocyanins; scopoletin (glycoalkaloid); Calcium oxalate.

Reasons to consume: The Doctrine of Signatures depicts the appearance of the pancreas was similar to a sweet potato. Consuming sweet potatoes can actually balance the glycemic index of diabetic individuals. Also know for the cholesterol balancing and vision supporting properties. These sweet potatoes come in different colors and their anthocyanins determine the pigment from white, yellow-orange, purple or violet. The purple and violet ones are supportive for cardiovascular health and arthritic conditions.

Reasons not to consume: Oxalates in the white and yellow versions need to be watched in individuals who have gout or rheumatic conditions.

ප ප ප

Daisy Composite Flower -- *Family Compositae*. Some of the most commonly consumed members are grouped below by their species.
- Lettuce (romaine, red leaf, green leaf, butter/bib)
- Chicory, endive, escarole, radicchio
- Globe artichoke
- Dandelion

High in Vitamins – Vitamin A, E and K in all members, Vitamin C in artichokes and romaine.

High in Minerals – Calcium, Magnesium.

Amino Acids Completeness – Daisy family members have an incomplete amino acid profile; other additional proteins need to be consumed to support necessary amino acid requirements in your diet.

Consumption Profile	Lettuce, Romaine 1 cup shred raw (47 g)	Chicory 1 cup chopped raw (29 g)	Escarole/ Endive ½ cup chopped raw (30 g)
Protein	0.6 g	0.6 g	0.3 g
Fat	0.1 g	0.1 g	0.0 g
Carbohydrates	1.5 g	1.4 g	0.8 g
Fiber	1.0 g	1.2 g	0.8 g

Consumption Profile	Artichoke 1 medium globe raw (128 g)	Dandelion 1 cup chopped raw (55 g)	Radicchio 1 cup shredded raw (40 g)
Protein	4.2 g	1.6 g	0.6 g
Fat	0.2 g	0.4 g	0.1 g
Carbohydrates	13.5 g	5.1 g	1.8 g
Fiber	6.9 g	1.9 g	0.4 g

Key Chemical components – Artichokes have *Solanine* (alkaloids) and cynarin (a liver supporting acid); all members have tannins; antioxidants; oxalates; inulin fiber.

Reasons to consume: Excellent for tonifying the body – highly alkaline food family. The bitter group of this family (chicory, radicchio, etc) are excellent for stimulating digestion. Also, members of this family of plants have diuretic benefits.

Reasons not to consume: Highly allergic plant family. Members of this family have cross reactions with other pollens to exacerbate symptoms. Consumption of these plants needs to be monitored, reduced or eliminated for those folks who are on anticoagulant therapy or have kidney, gout or rheumatic conditions.

೮೮ ೮೮ ೮೮

Gourd -- *Family Cucurbitaceae*: Cucurbits is the more accurate name for this family and its members. It is split into three main groups: Squashes, melons and gourds. The following is a list of the more commonly consumed members of two of the groups:
- Crookneck squash, butternut squash, acorn squash, spaghetti squash (winter Squashes), pumpkin, summer squash
- Melons
    o Watermelon
    o Cantaloupe
    o Honeydew
    o Cucumber

High in Vitamins – Vitamin A in cantaloupe, Vitamin C in all in varying levels, Choline.

High in Minerals – Calcium, Potassium, Lithium.

Amino Acids Completeness – Gourds/Cucurbits have an incomplete amino acid profile; other additional proteins need to be consumed to support necessary amino acid requirements in your diet.

Consumption Profile	Cantaloupe 1 cup raw (177 g)	Honeydew 1 cup raw (177 g)	Watermelon 1 cup raw (154 g)
Protein	1.5 g	1.0 g	0.9 g
Fat	0.3 g	0.2 g	0.2 g
Carbohydrates	15.6 g	16.1 g	11.6 g
Fiber	1.6 g	1.4 g	0.0 g

Consumption Profile	Cucumber with skin, raw ½ cup sliced (52 g)	Pumpkin 1 cup cubes raw (116 g)	Squashes – Winter / Summer 1 cup raw (116 g)
Protein	0.3 g	1.2 g	1.1 - 1.4 g
Fat	0.1 g	0.1 g	0.2 g
Carbohydrates	1.9 g	7.5 g	3.8 – 10.0g summer – winter
Fiber	0.3 g	0.6 g	1.2 - 1.7 g summer - winter

Key Chemical components – Most of these plant members have an even (1:1) to 3:1 ratio of Omega-3 to Omega-6, except for watermelon which only has Omega-6. Phytosterols – Erepsine; cellulose.

Reasons to consume: Alkaline foods family members which are excellent for maintaining our health. This food family has antibacterial, anticancer, anticoagulant, and antioxidant properties. These plant members also have properties to balance the intestinal flora (Erepsine) and keep the colon clean. Additionally, this family is known for its topically applied supportive skin benefits (antioxidant) – oily/uneven skin, burns, and wrinkles.

Reasons not to consume: This family of plants are known for increasing the amount of intestinal mucous. As such these family members are not the best for delicate stomachs, or those who have diarrhea frequently. We need to chew these foods well or else the high cellulose content will not be broken down enough to support digestion.

CB CB CB

Yam -- *Family Dioscoreaceae*: This is more a traditional tuber in structure compared to a sweet potato (Convolvulaceae). This tuber has different origins and drier, starchier texture.

High in Vitamins – Vitamin C and K.

High in Minerals – Potassium.

Amino Acids Completeness – Yams have an incomplete amino acid profile; other additional proteins need to be consumed to support necessary amino acid requirements in your diet.

Consumption Profile	Yam – 1 cup cubed raw (150 g)
Protein	2.3 g
Fat	0.3 g
Carbohydrates	41.8 g
Fiber	6.1 g

Key Chemical components – Yam has salicylate properties, (similar components to aspirin) of an analgesic nature; and oxalates. Additionally it has an estrogenic saponin – Diosgenin. This plant has Omega-3 & 6 – 1:4.25 ratio of Omega-3 to Omega 6.

Reasons to consume: Lower in calories than its misnomer of a food cousin, sweet potato; has diuretic, cholesterol reducing cardiovascular and arthritic benefits as well as hormone support for menopause (all from the Diosgenin).

Reasons not to consume: Consumption needs to be monitored for those who have Salicylates sensitivity. Diosgenin is reduced when the yam is cooked, however over-consumption of this plant can promote toxicity reactions. If pregnant, it is wise to avoid consumption or keep to minimum to prevent estrogen triggered contractions. Also consuming this plant may enhance any medical cholesterol therapy in place and needs to be monitored.

CB CB CB

Heath/Bilberry -- *Family Ericaceae*: Blueberry and cranberry are two of the key fruits from this plant family. Blueberries are more of a mountain shrub while the cranberry shrubs are grown in the wetlands.

High in Vitamins – Vitamin C in both; Vitamin E in blueberries.

High in Minerals – Manganese.

Amino Acids Completeness – Heath family members have an incomplete amino acid profile; other additional proteins need to be consumed to support necessary amino acid requirements in your diet.

Consumption Profile	Blueberry, Wild 1 cup raw (148 g)	Cranberry 1 cup chopped raw (110 g)
Protein	1.1 g	0.4 g
Fat	0.5 g	0.1 g
Carbohydrates	21.4 g	13.4 g
Fiber	3.6 g	5.4 g

Key Chemical components – Omega-3 & 6 with 1:15 ratio of Omega-3 to Omega-6; anthocyanins; salicylic acid; antioxidants; ellagic acid, hippuric acid; caffeic acid, gallic acid, hydroquinone; quercetin, Rutin; kaempferol, chlorogenic acid; solanine (in blueberries).

Reasons to consume: Both blueberries and cranberries have a chemical – hippuric acid which helps with the kidneys and bladder to help relieve infections through changing the pH of the urine. Additionally the juice of these members helps in the break down of oxalates and kidney stones. These family members have digestive and ocular benefits as well. Bottom line – this food family and its antibacterial, antioxidant and anti-viral strengths make this a must have in your diet.

Reasons not to consume: Blueberries have *solanine* in their skin similar to potatoes. It is best to eat the darkest, ripest blueberries to avoid any solanine related stomach upset/issues. Folks who are sensitive to salicylic acid will need to monitor their reactions as there is a significant amount found in cranberries.

 C3 C3 C3

Laurel -- *Family Lauraceae*: Two of the most unlikely plants are members of the same family, avocado and cinnamon. What is it about the Laurel family that could produce two vastly different members?

High in Vitamins – Vitamin K, D, E, Folate.

High in Minerals – Potassium in avocado; Manganese in cinnamon.

Amino Acids Completeness – Laurel family members have a complete amino acid profile; no additional proteins need to be consumed to support necessary amino acid requirements in your diet.

Consumption Profile	Avocado, California 1 c pureed raw (230 g)	Cinnamon 1 tsp (8 g)
Protein	4.5 g	0.3 g
Fat	35.4 g	0.1 g
Carbohydrates	19.9 g	6.2 g
Fiber	15.6 g	4.1 g

Key Chemical components – Omega-3 & 6 – Higher Omega-3 than 6; Saponins; Lecithin; Phytosterols; caretenoids; epicatechins; glutathione (in avocado).

Reasons to consume: Avocados has a key similarities to the female reproductive system (an avocado is shaped like a uterus and takes 9 months to mature, just like a human baby). Avocado have therapeutic aspects in maintaining a woman's reproductive health by balancing their hormones and protecting against cervical cancers. Additionally, consuming avocado daily helps with the maintenance and control of cholesterol levels. The glutathione helps to lower the serum and LDL cholesterol and acts as a vasodilator.

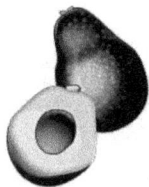

Cinnamon has antiviral properties. One-half teaspoon daily helps support our immune balance. Additionally, cinnamon is excellent at regulating our sugar balance in the bloodstream. It also has analgesic and anticoagulant properties.

Reasons not to consume: Avocados are too high in fats. There is no reason not to eat cinnamon ☺. True cinnamon (not the Cassia substitute) does not have high levels of coumarin in it, which would make it something to monitor and limit consumption for those on Warfarin/Coumadin therapy.

08 08 08

Pomegranate -- *Family Lythraceae.* This family is the sister of the Myrtle family. Pomegranates are only available for 5 months out of the year. So when they are in season, nothing beats this phytonutrient packed unique fruit.

High in Vitamins –Folate and Choline.

High in Minerals – Copper.

Amino Acids Completeness – Pomegranates have an incomplete amino acid profile; additional other proteins need to be consumed to support necessary amino acid requirements in your diet.

Consumption Profile	Pomegranate 1 – 4 inch diameter (282 g)
Protein	4.7 g
Fat	3.3 g
Carbohydrates	52.7 g
Fiber	11.3 g

Key Chemical components – Omega-6; anthocyanin; tannins; polyphenols; punicalagins; insoluble fiber

Reasons to consume: Help maintain cardiovascular health and reduce free radicals through the antioxidant compounds (anthocyanin and punicalagins). This member has hypotensive and diuretic properties along with its fiber benefits.

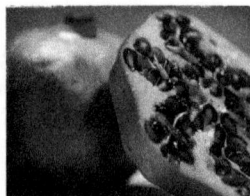

Reasons not to consume: In the case of diarrhea, this food would be contraindicated. This would exacerbate the condition, releasing more fluid and electrolytes

 C3 C3 C3

Cola Nut -- *Family Malvaceae*: Chocolate, Cacao, Cocoa, and Okra. Bet you did not see that coming – *Chocolate* and *Okra* in the same family. Both have interesting nutritional benefits that are shared and those unique to each of them.

High in Vitamins – Vitamin K, C and Folate in okra; No high vitamins in cocoa.

High in Minerals – Manganese in both; Copper, Magnesium, Iron, Phosphorus in cocoa; Calcium and Potassium in okra.

Amino Acids Completeness – Cola nut family members have an incomplete amino acid profile; other additional proteins need to be consumed to support necessary amino acid requirements in your diet.

Consumption Profile	Cocoa Unsweetened Dry powder 1 cup (86 g)	Okra 1 cup (100 g)
Protein	16.9 g	2.0 g
Fat	11.8 g	0.1 g
Carbohydrates	49.8 g	7.0 g
Fiber	28.5 g	3.2 g

Key Chemical components – Therbromine in cocoa; Catechins, Tannins; mucilage / fiber in Okra; Gossypol in okra seeds (contraceptive).

Reasons to consume: The catechins/tannins in these food family members reduce oxidative stress in our bodies. This antioxidant effect can lower chances of heart disease. Okra is known for its mucilaginous content and diuretic properties. The glutathione in okra makes it a great free radical reducing, cardiovascular supporting and vasodilating food.

Reasons not to consume: Cocoa is alkaline on its own; when processed with dairy to make candy, it loses its alkalinity. The Therbromine is a toxic alkaloid in large quantities. Your pets (dogs, cats, bird and horses) can be poisoned easily by a small amount of cocoa/cacao or chocolate. Okra seeds have a contraceptive compound which is used to control sperm.

CB CB CB

Mulberry -- *Family Moraceae*: Mulberry and fig are the two key members of this family. If you look closely to these two fruits you will find an interesting relationship. The mulberry fruit is similar to an inside-out version of the fig. Also, this plant family is a sister branch to the ***Rosaceae*** (Rose) family.

High in Vitamins – Vitamin C, A.

High in Minerals – Iron, Potassium.

Amino Acids Completeness – Mulberries and figs have an incomplete amino acid profile; other additional proteins need to be consumed to support necessary amino acid requirements in your diet.

Consumption Profile	Mulberry 1 cup raw (140 g)	Fig 1 large 2.5 in diameter raw (64 g)
Protein	2.0 g	0.5 g
Fat	0.5 g	0.2 g
Carbohydrates	13.7 g	12.3 g
Fiber	2.4 g	1.9 g

Key Chemical components – Omega-3 & 6 (in fig only Omega-6); pectins; flavonoids; gallic acid, chlorogenic acid, syringic acid, catechin, epicatechin and rutin; reservatrol; enzymes (Esterase, Ficin, Fucomarine), Beta-carotene.

Reasons to consume: According to the Doctrine of Signatures, figs support male fertility. Figs grow in pairs and are full of seeds, just like in the male anatomy. Figs have native anticancer properties from the beta-carotene.

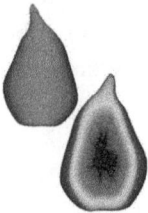

Reasons not to consume: This family has been known to react with the Latex-Fruit Allergy. Also, handling the raw fruits can promote photo sensitivity (fucomarine enzyme).

CB CB CB

Banana -- *Family Musaceae*: Banana and plantain are not really different genetic members of this family. Plantain is a hybrid of the 'sweet banana' species which possesses more starchy flesh.

High in Vitamins – Vitamin B6, C, Choline and Betaine are in both. Plantain has added Vitamin A.

High in Minerals – Potassium in both members. Manganese and Fluoride is found in bananas only.

Amino Acids Completeness – Bananas and Plantains have an incomplete amino acid profile; other additional proteins need to be consumed to support necessary amino acid requirements in your diet.

Consumption Profile	Banana 1 cup mashed raw (225 g)	Plantains 1 cup sliced raw (148 g)
Protein	2.5 g	1.9 g
Fat	0.7 g	0.5 g
Carbohydrates	51.4 g	47.2 g
Fiber	5.9 g	3.4 g

Key Chemical components – Omega-3 & 6 in close ratio of 1:2. Chemical compound which prevent ulcers in these family members; fiber; tannins.

Reasons to consume: Anti-ulcer benefits in both members. The flesh helps to heal the damaged area and when consumed regularly acts as a preventative therapy. They also have dietary stimulant and astringent properties. The potassium in these members is excellent for helping to eliminate extra fluids to maintain our bodies' water/sodium balance. Rubbing the skin of the banana or plantain on skin afflictions or warts can facilitate their healing due to the antibacterial/antiviral components.

Reasons not to consume: There has been documented cross sensitivity between banana family members with rubber and latex allergies. This sensitivity can be exhibited as mildly as Oral Allergy Syndrome or as dangerous as anaphylactic IgE. Also, those who have issues with liver functioning, and cardiac arrhythmias should avoid or limit consumption of these food family members. The potassium facilitates the water/sodium balance towards removing excess fluids. This can impact those which cardiovascular issues.

ೞ   ೞ   ೞ

Olive -- *Family Oleaceae*. Green and black olives are a focal point in the Mediterranean diet. As more information is shared about the essential fatty acid benefits, more folks are trying these as snacks, adding them into salads and cooking with them.

High in Vitamins – Choline.

High in Minerals – Sodium, Chlorine.

Amino Acids Completeness – Olives have an incomplete amino acid profile; other additional proteins need to be consumed to support necessary amino acid requirements in your diet.

Consumption Profile	Green Olive pickled, canned (100 g)	Black Olive Ripe, canned (100 g)
Protein	1.0 g	0.8
Fat	15.3 g	10.7 g
Carbohydrates	3.8 g	6.3 g
Fiber	3.3 g	3.2 g

Key Chemical components – High in Omega-3 and 6 essential fatty acids. Ratio is high in Omega-6 versus Omega-3; phenolic compounds – hydroxytyrosol to name one and glycoside/terpine – oleuropein; cellulose; pectins; lignin; hydroxycinnamic acids, flavonols; and anthocyanins.

Reasons to consume: Olive oil is one of the few oils that is beneficial to consume due to the essential fatty acid compounds. Olives and their essential fatty acids are

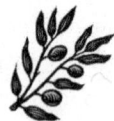

supportive of female reproductive organs as they look like the ovaries. For a small drupe – it has antioxidant, anti-inflammatory and anticancer properties; this is one of the most highly packed phytonutrient food families known.

Reasons not to consume: As a consumable plant, these family members are high in fat and sodium. Even olive oil is high in fat, based on calories and should be consumed in moderation.

 C8 C8 C8

Buckwheat -- *Family Polygonaceae*: Plants in this family are buckwheat, rhubarb, and sorrel. Rhubarb and sorrel will be discussed here.

High in Vitamins – Reasonably high Vitamin K, A and C and Choline

High in Minerals – Sorrel is reasonably high in calcium, magnesium, niacin, and riboflavin. Rhubarb has the same minerals, just not as high a concentration as sorrel.

Amino Acids Completeness – Buckwheat family members have an incomplete amino acid profile; other additional proteins need to be consumed to support necessary amino acid requirements in your diet.

Consumption Profile	Rhubarb 1 c diced (122 g)	Sorrel ½ cup
Protein	1.1 g	1.3 g
Fat	0.2 g	2.1 g
Carbohydrates	5.5 g	0.5 g
Fiber	2.2 g	1.9 g

Key Chemical components – Flavonoids; Anthocyanins; Anthraquinones; fiber; Oxalic Acid.

Reasons to consume: Rhubarb relieves constipation and blocks excess sugar. The anthraquinones found in rhubarb are shown to prevent cancer in the body. Sorrel's flavonoids have been shown to help kidney function as a diuretic, and reduce risk of certain cancers.

Reasons not to consume: Rhubarb and sorrel is consumed cooked. Sorrel can be consume in liquid form as sorrel water. Both family members have high levels of oxalic acid (especially in the leaves of the rhubarb which are **not to be eaten**). The oxalic acid may exacerbate episodes of gout, kidney stones or rheumatism. It is also a natural laxative. Be careful not to over-consume in either form. Also do not cook sorrel in aluminum as it leaches the metal from the pot into the cooked product.

ଔ ଔ ଔ

Rose -- *Family Rosaceae*: This food family is one that is frequently consumed by humans and animals alike. This is a complicated family with multiple branches which document their differences in their specific types of fruits. The main part of the family has blackberry, boysenberry, raspberry, and rosehip. Strawberries are in their own sub-family within Rose family. Otherwise, there are two sub-families which have been know to delineate specific and potential allergies and sensitivities.

Prune/Plum -- *Sub Family Amygdaloideae*: These are the stone fruit sub group of the Rose family which is broken into two specific types:

- Genus Prunoideae - Plum, prune, cherry, nectarine, apricot, pluot, and peach

- Genus Maloideae - Apple, pear

These two subfamily-genus groups hold the most frequently consumed fruits.

High in Vitamins – Vitamin C, Vitamin K.

High in Minerals – Manganese, Fluoride, Lithium.

Amino Acids Completeness – Rose family members have an incomplete amino acid profile; other additional proteins need to be consumed to support necessary amino acid requirements in your diet.

Consumption Profile	Blackberry 1 cup raw (144 g)	Raspberry 1 cup raw (123g)	Strawberries 1 c halves (152 g)
Protein	2.0 g	1.5 g	1.0 g
Fat	0.7 g	0.8 g	0.5 g
Carbohydrates	14.7 g	14.7 g	11.7 g
Fiber	7.6 g	8.0 g	3.0 g

Consumption Profile	Plum 1 cup raw sliced (165 g)	Peach 1 raw large 2.75 in diameter (175 g)	Cherry 1 cup with pits (138 g)
Protein	1.2 g	1.6 g	1.5 g
Fat	0.5 g	0.4 g	0.3 g
Carbohydrates	18.8 g	17.3 g	22.1 g
Fiber	2.3 g	2.6 g	2.9 g

Consumption Profile	Apricot 1 cup halves (125 g)	Apple 1 cup raw chopped (125 g)	Pear 1 raw small (148 g)
Protein	2.2 g	0.3 g	0.6 g
Fat	0.6 g	0.2 g	0.2 g
Carbohydrates	17.4 g	17.3 g	22.9 g
Fiber	3.1 g	3.0 g	4.6 g

Key Chemical components – Members of the Rose family, Prune sub-family possess a glycoside called Amygdalin. This is found in the seed of the stone fruits. They also possess phytonutrients (tannin, catechin, ellagic acid), salicylates, polyphenols and Omega-3 & 6 essential fatty acids. Apples have solanine as well though not as much as in the Nightshade family. It is present when the apples are maturing.

Reasons to consume: Members of this food family have antibacterial, antioxidant, antiviral and anticancer properties. Additionally they have cholesterol lowering and cardiovascular supporting properties. Members of this family are considered acidic foods and should be consumed in moderation.

Reasons not to consume: It is unwise to eat the seeds of this family of plants, on a consistent basis, since they contain Amygdalin. A specific enzyme (beta-glucosidase) in the gut can release the cyanide component of the amygdalin into the body resulting in poisoning. Those who are solanine sensitive should avoid eating granny smith apples and those apples which have not completely matured (no green tint) to them. Additionally those who are sensitive to salicylates should be monitoring, reducing or avoiding these family members.

Ↄ Ↄ Ↄ

Madder -- *Family Rubiaceae*: This family possesses one of the most addictive plants that are consumed every day – coffee. This fruit when roasted and brewed is the morning beverage of choice for many.

High in Vitamins – None.

High in Minerals – Potassium.

Amino Acids Completeness – Coffee has an incomplete amino acid profile; other additional proteins need to be consumed to support necessary amino acid requirements in your diet.

Consumption Profile	Coffee roasted ground, brewed with tap water 1 cup (237 g)
Protein	0.3 o
Fat	0.0 g
Carbohydrates	0.0 g
Fiber	0.0 g

Key Chemical components – Glycoalkaloid (Caffeine); Tannins

Reasons to consume: Caffeine is a nervous system stimulant, vasodilator and diuretic. This can be helpful in improving metabolic performance. The antioxidant properties of the roasted coffee bean are helpful in preventing free radicals from damaging the body. Also, the caffeine in coffee can be used as an antidepressant as it affects the dopamine reaction, reducing feelings of depression.

Reasons not to consume: Tannins, caffeine, and pesticides in commercially grown beans. Excess coffee consumption can negatively impact LDL cholesterol level, increase anxiety, increase intensity of headaches and lead to anemia. The polyphenols in coffee can block absorption of Iron. The best recommendation to balance the benefits and risks of consumption is *moderation.*

ଔ ଔ ଔ

Citrus -- *Family Rutaceae:* One of the most commonly consumed food families whose members have a higher likelihood of food allergy and sensitivity. The primary citrus family members are grapefruit, lemon, lime, orange, and tangerine.

High in Vitamins – Vitamin C (in most of these members); Vitamin K in grapefruit, Vitamin A in oranges and lemons.

High in Minerals – Potassium.

Amino Acids Completeness – Citrus family members have an incomplete amino acid profile; other additional proteins need to be consumed to support necessary amino acid requirements in your diet.

Consumption Profile	Grapefruit raw 1 cup (230 g)	Orange raw, 1 cup (170 g)	Tangerine raw, 1 cup sections (195 g)
Protein	1.6 g	2.2 g	1.6 g
Fat	0.2 g	0.5 g	0.6 g
Carbohydrates	19.3 g	26.3 g	26.3 g
Fiber	2.5 g	7.7 g	3.5 g

Consumption Profile	Lemon raw 1 fruit no seeds (108 g)	Lime raw 1 fruit (67 g)
Protein	1.3 g	0.5 g
Fat	0.3 g	0.1 g
Carbohydrates	11.6 g	7.1 g
Fiber	5.1 g	1.9 g

Key Chemical components – Bioflavonoids; antibacterial properties in the Grapefruit seed; Omega-3 & 6 though slightly higher in the 6. Phytosterols; Hesperitin, Hesperidin; Diosmin; Inositol (except in Lemons); Naringin; Rutin.

Reasons to consume: Lemon, though acidic in nature, turns alkaline in our bodies. One of the best things to have first thing in the morning is fresh lemon tea – juice of half a lemon in hot water. The antioxidants in grapefruits have been shown to lower serum cholesterol and triglycerides. The hesperidin/hesperitin/diosmin content in these food family members have anti-viral and antihistamine properties. These elements are also good

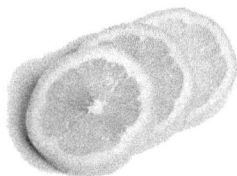

for reducing edema. According to the Doctrine of Signatures, members of the citrus family mimic the mammary glands of females. These fruits are supportive of breast health and lymphatic drainage in and out of the tissues.

Reasons not to consume: This food family is very acidic in nature. The frequent consumption of these plants can erode the enamel on your teeth. Additionally, this a family which can trigger the Oral Allergy Syndrome and also other skin related allergic reactions. Grapefruits are known to interfere with commercial medicines for high blood pressure and clotting.

෬   ෬   ෬

Carrot -- *Family Umbelliferae*: Members of this family are parsley, parsnip, carrot, celery, celeriac, and fennel. This predominately root based plant family has many antioxidant benefits.

High in Vitamins – Vitamin A, B6 found in carrots and parsley; Vitamin C found in parsley; Vitamin K found in parsley and celeriac.

High in Minerals – Sodium found in celery.

Amino Acids Completeness – Carrot family members have an incomplete amino acid profile; additional other proteins need to be consumed to support necessary amino acid requirements in your diet.

Consumption Profile	Carrot 1 cup raw (128 g)	Parsley 1 cup raw (60 g)	Parsnip 1 cup sliced raw (133 g)
Protein	1.2 g	1.8 g	1.0 g
Fat	0.3 g	0.5 g	0.4 g
Carbohydrates	12.3 g	3.8 g	23.9 g
Fiber	3.6 g	2.0 g	6.5 g

Consumption Profile	Celery 1 cup raw (101 g)	Celeriac 1 cup raw (156 g)	Fennel 1 cup raw (87 g)
Protein	0.7 g	2.3 g	1.1 g
Fat	0.2 g	0.5 g	0.2 g
Carbohydrates	3.5 g	14.4 g	6.3 g
Fiber	1.6 g	2.8 g	2.7 g

Key Chemical components – Phytosterols; Omega-3 & 6 though slightly higher in Omega-6 than 3; antioxidants; flavonoids; fiber; stimulating volatile oils; oxalic acid (in Parsley).

Reasons to consume: According to the Doctrine of Signatures, Carrots and their relative parsnip are supportive to eye health. When you slice a carrot parallel to the root, you can see the plant resembles an eye. Vitamin A found in these family members is known for supporting our eyes. Vitamin A supports the blood flow to the eyes and helps with maintaining healthy eye functions.

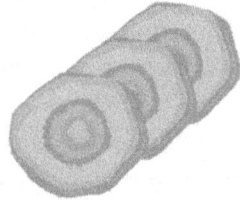

Celery looks like the bones of the body and has the same percentage of sodium as our bones. If the sodium is not properly regulated it pulls the sodium from the bones which weakens them. Celery also has calcium and silica which help maintain the integrity of our bone structure.

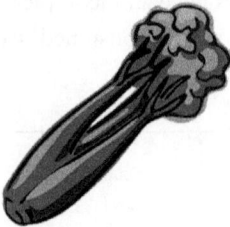

The stimulating volatile oils from this food family key components to their antibacterial, anti-inflammatory, antioxidant and anticancer activities. The oils shut down the tumor necrosis factor and prevents altering of cells.

Reasons not to consume: Carrots and Parsnips are high on the glycemic index (high in natural sugars). Members of this family produce a sodium storing effect and that can result in higher blood pressure and edema. Additionally, parsley should be consumed in moderation by those folks who have kidney issues (oxalic acid).

C
CB CB CB

Grape -- *Family Vitaceae*: Some of these family's members are grape, currants, and raisin. This family is a contributor to many derivative products; wines, champagne, food coloring, and vinegars to name a key few.

High in Vitamins – Grapes are high in Vitamin C & K; Vitamin C in currants is high.

High in Minerals – Grapes are high in Manganese; Currants have it, just not in a large quantity.

Amino Acids Completeness – Grapes and currants have an incomplete amino acid profile; other additional proteins need to be consumed to support necessary amino acid requirements in your diet.

Consumption Profile	Currants European Black, raw 1 cup (112 g)	Grapes American type, raw, slip skin 1 cup (92 g)
Protein	1.6 g	0.6 g
Fat	0.5 g	0.3 g
Carbohydrates	17.2 g	15.8 g
Fiber	2.0 g	0.8 g

Key Chemical components – Proanthocyanin, a condensed form of tannins; bioflavonoids; hydroxybenzoic acids; reservatrol; ellagic acid, caffeic acid; oxalates (in concord/dark grapes and currants).

Reasons to consume: Grapes resemble the alveoli in our lungs in the way that they grow in clumps. Consuming grapes as part of the diet can reduce the chance of getting lung cancer and emphysema. The proanthocyanin found in the grape seeds may lower the intensity of an allergy triggered asthma attack. These plant members have anticoagulant, anti-viral and

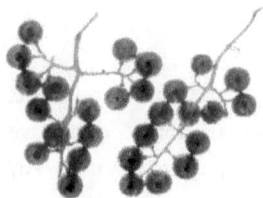

antioxidant properties. As an alkaline food family, these members are excellent for removing toxins when consumed almost exclusively. The best time to perform this food detox during the peak of harvest season (late Summer).

Reasons not to consume: Consumption of these plants needs to be monitored, reduced or eliminated for those folks who are on anticoagulant therapy or have kidney, gout or rheumatic conditions. The oxalates levels are less in the green grapes and those are better to consume. If you have diabetic conditions, it would be wise to reduce/avoid this family altogether from the high sugar content.

cs cs cs

Ginger -- *Family Zingiberaceae*. - Ginger is the key member of this family to be discussed. This plant is more than the herb classification. Ginger is a plant with many medicinal qualities. It has analgesic, anticancer, anticoagulant, antioxidant, anti-viral and sedative properties.

High in Vitamins – None.

High in Minerals – None.

Amino Acids Completeness – Ginger has an incomplete amino acid profile; other additional proteins need to be consumed to support necessary amino acid requirements in your diet.

Consumption Profile	Ginger – raw ¼ cup slices (24 g)
Protein	0.1 g
Fat	0.2 g
Carbohydrates	4.3 g
Fiber	0.5 g

Key Chemical components – Phytosterols; oxalic acid; Omega-3 & 6; essential oils (ginerol); cucurmin; fiber; digestive enzyme – zingibain; salicylates; polyphenols.

Reasons to consume: As per the Doctrine of Signatures, ginger mimics the structure of the stomach. It is used to tonify and comfort upset stomach and nausea. This root has been used for motion sickness and to aid digestion for thousands of years. Its carminative properties help expel gas from the gastrointestinal tract. This plant and its family members also have anti-inflammatory, antibacterial, analgesic, anticoagulant, antioxidant, and sedative properties.

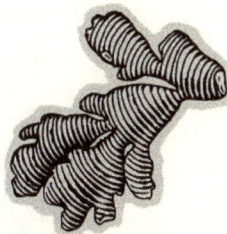

Reasons not to consume: This plant should be used with caution by pregnant women as the compounds could potentially induce abortion. Also Monitoring of consumption is needed when consumed by individuals who are on blood thinners because the compounds may interfere with vitamin / mineral absorption. The curcumin in these family members may product phototoxic reactions when exposed to excessive amounts/high concentrations of sunlight. Inhaling the dried ground ginger plant may produce an IgE allergic response.

Food Combination – FRUITS & VEGETABLES

Remember to consult the "Dirty Dozen" (See Chapter 11 for list) and top 15 clean fruits and vegetables when purchasing and preparing for your meal. If you bought one of the "Dirty Dozen", please make sure to wash thoroughly and peel if able to ensure removal of pesticides.

Most fruits and vegetable process through the digestive system in 1 – 2 hours. Fruits are always best consumed alone and no more than 2 or 3 fruits together from the same acid/alkaline group. When combined with non starchy vegetables– digestion is enhanced; when combined with starchy vegetables then it can take *longer* (between 2 and 3 hours) for the stomach to empty due to the extra digestion processing.

The following plants and/or animals are evaluated to combine with fruits**
& vegetables:

Excellent – Non-starchy vegetables go well with everything
Good – Mildly starchy vegetables can be combined with animal proteins &
dairy, grasses & grains, starchy vegetables, legumes
Poor – None

** Some of the commonly consumed fruits are grouped as follows:

Acid Fruits	Sub Acid Fruits	Sweet Fruits	Melon
Blackberry	Apple	Banana	Cantaloupe
Grapefruit	Apricot	Dates	Casaba Melon
Lemon/Lime	Blueberry	Currants	Crenshaw Melon
Orange	Cherry	Figs	Honeydew Melon
Pineapple	Kiwi	Grapes	Persian Melon
Plum (Sour)	Mango	Papaya	Watermelon
Pomegranate	Peach	Persimmon	
Raspberry	Pear	Prunes	
Sour Apple	Plum (Sweet)	Raisins	
Strawberry			

Pollen interactions when consuming fruits & vegetables

Can inhaling specific pollens exacerbate allergic or sensitive reaction to
foods consumed? Additionally, can having a specific condition increase the
sensitivity or reactions to food? Dr. Jacqueline Krohn and other physicians
have documented examples of these occurrences:

Pollen	*Food Family/Members*
Cottonwood Pollen, Mugwort Pollen and Ragweed Pollen	*Compositae - Lettuce*
Elm Pollen, Ragweed Pollen and Viral Infections	*Labiatae – Mint*
Oak Pollen, Mugwort Pollen and Birch Pollen; Latex-Fruit Allergy	*Rosaceae – Rose*
Pecan Pollen, Hickory Pollen and Ragweed Pollen; Dust Mite Allergy, Latex-Fruit Allergy	*Musaceae – Banana*

Sage Pollen, Birch Pollen and Mugwort Pollens	*Umbrelliferaceae - Parsley*
Ragweed Pollen, Mugwort Pollen, and Birch Pollen; Latex-Fruit Allergy	*Cucurbitaceae – Melons*
Viral Infections	*Liliaceae – Lily*
Dust Mite Allergy, Latex-Fruit Allergy; Birch Pollen and Mugwort Pollen	*Actinidiacea – Kiwi*
Latex-Fruit Allergy	*Zingiberaceae - Ginger*
Latex-Fruit Allergy	*Bromeliaceae - Pineapple*
Latex-Fruit Allergy	*Anacardiaceae - Mango*
Latex-Fruit Allergy	*Caricaceae - Papaya*

Also the following are key food combinations that may increase the risk of reactivity for specific fruits & vegetables:

- Corn and banana
- Egg and apple
- Cane Sugar and orange
- Milk and mint
- Wheat and tea
- Chocolate and coffee
- Milk and chocolate
- Cola and chocolate
- Cola and coffee

Blood Type Impacts

In **Eat Right for your Type**, Dr. Peter D'Adamo documents the reactions of food to one's health, based on Blood Type (and GenoType). If you follow the specifics below for A or B blood types and still have issues, you may be a mixed blood type (part A or B and part O). Please refer to the Let's Get Started section to review for more information about mixed blood types. It would be best to evaluate both blood types' food specifics and see where your reactions lie.

Fruits to Avoid by Blood Type

O	A	B	AB
Apple Cider/Juice	Banana	Avocado	Avocado
Avocado	Cantaloupe	Coconut Water/Milk	Banana
Blackberry/Blackberry Juice	Coconut Water/Milk	Persimmon	Coconut Water/Milk
Cantaloupe	Honeydew	Pomegranate	Guava
Coconut Water/Milk	Mango/Mango Juice	Prickly Pear	Mango/Mango Juice
Honeydew	Orange/Orange Juice	Starfruit (Carambola)	Persimmon
Mango/Mango Juice	Papaya/		Pomegranate
Orange/Orange Juice	Papaya Juice		Prickly Pear
Plantain	Plantain		Starfruit (Carambola)
Strawberry	Tangerine/Tangerine Juice		
Tangerine/Tangerine Juice			

Fruits that are Beneficial by Blood Type

O	A	B	AB
Banana	Apricot/Apricot Juice	Banana	Cherry (Bing, Sweet, White, etc)
Blueberry	Blackberry/Blackberry Juice	Cranberry	Black Cherry Juice
Black Cherry (Juice)	Blueberry	Cranberry Juice	Cranberry
Fig (Fresh or Dried)	Boysenberry	Grape	Cranberry Juice
Guava	Cherry (Bing, Sweet, White, etc)	Papaya	Fig (Fresh or Dried)
Mango	Black Cherry Juice	Papaya Juice	Gooseberry
Pineapple Juice	Cranberry	Pineapple	Grape
Plum (Dark/Green/Red)	Grapefruit/Grapefruit Juice	Pineapple Juice	Grapefruit
Prune/Prune Juice	Lemon/Lemon Juice	Plum (Dark/Green/Red)	Kiwi
	Pineapple		Lemon/Lemon Juice
	Pineapple Juice		Loganberry
	Plum (Dark/Green/Red)		Papaya Juice
	Prune/Prune Juice		Pineapple
	Raisin		Plum (Dark/Green/Red)
	Water + Lemon		

Vegetables to Avoid by Blood Type

O	A	B	AB
Alfalfa Sprouts	Cabbage(Chinese/Red/White)	Aloe/Aloe Tea/Aloe Juice	Aloe/Aloe Tea/Aloe Juice
Aloe/Aloe Tea/Aloe Juice	Caper	Artichoke	Artichoke
Brussel Sprout	Olive (Black)	Olive (Black)	Caper
Cabbage(Chinese/Red/White)	Olive (Greek/Spanish)	Olive (Greek/Spanish)	Olive (Black)
Cabbage Juice	Potato (Sweet)	Olive (Green)	Pickle
Caper	Rhubarb	Pumpkin	Radish
Cauliflower	Sauerkraut	Radish	Radish Sprouts
Mustard Greens	Yam	Radish Sprouts	Rhubarb
Olive (Black)		Rhubarb	
Olive (Greek/Spanish)			
Pickle			
Rhubarb			
Sauerkraut			
Spirulina /Spirulina Juice			

Vegetables that are Beneficial by Blood Type

O	A	B	AB
Artichoke	Alfalfa Sprouts	Beet	Alfalfa Sprouts
Beet Greens	Aloe/Aloe Tea/Aloe Juice	Beet Greens	Beet
Broccoli	Artichoke	Beet Juice	Beet Greens
Chicory	Beet Greens	Broccoli	Beet Juice
Collard Greens	Broccoli	Brussel Sprouts	Broccoli
Dandelion	Carrot	Cabbage (Chinese/Red/White)	Cabbage Juice
Escarole	Carrot Juice	Cabbage Juice	Carrot Juice
Garlic	Celery Juice	Carrot	Cauliflower
Horseradish	Chicory	Cauliflower	Celery
Kale	Collard Greens	Collard Greens	Celery Juice
Kelp	Dandelion	Ginger	Collard Greens
Kohlrabi	Escarole	Kale	Cucumber
Leek	Garlic	Mustard Greens	Dandelion
Lettuce (Romaine)	Ginger	Parsnip	Garlic
Okra	Horseradish	Potato (Sweet)	Kale
Onion (Red/Spanish/Yellow)	Kale	Yam	Mustard Greens
Parsnip	Kohlrabi		Parsnip
Potato (Sweet)	Leek		Potato (Sweet)

Pumpkin	Lettuce (Romaine)		Yam
Seaweed	Okra		
Spinach/ Spinach Juice	Onion (Red/Spanish/Yellow)		
Swiss Chard	Parsnip		
Turnip	Pumpkin		
	Spinach/Spinach Juice		
	Swiss Chard		
	Turnip		

All other fruits and vegetables not listed in tables have a neutral impact by blood types.

In general, Blood Type O is the most susceptible to fruit and vegetable allergies and intolerances. This is due to the meat-eating (hunter) origins of this blood type.

General Foodergies™ Issues

As you can see this is by far the largest section of the book – so many plant families! Due to the nature of plants, the likelihood of food family allergy and sensitivity issues is higher than with animal proteins.

There are differences in species which can delineate members of a family that may be consumed versus others, like in the case of the Rose family members; you may be allergic or have sensitivity to the entire family or just one branch. For example, the Prunus sub group, where almonds come from may be your issue or maybe just the side where apples exist.

Another case would be in specific members of the Cruciferous vegetables – where consuming some of them (broccoli or arugula) is fine and others (cabbage or brussels sprouts) presents a digestive challenge.

If you have specific questions about members of a food family or if a food is not listed in this book (in the detailed chapters or the reference in Chapter 3), please ask your question via the Foodergies™! Community Forum (http://foodergies.forumcommunity.net), subscribe to my blog at www.keileswellnesscare.com, or send email to **foodergies@gmail.com**.

11 SUPPORTING DOCUMENTS & LINKS

With all the information, it is important to share some sample documents to facilitate your own data collection. The following lists the forms, references to charts and quizzes used by me from other sources and with my clients in the investigation of their food families.

Online additional food family reference: This will be the web page for the updates to the food family details not included in this book.
http://www.keileswellnesscare.com/foodfamilysummary.html

Links to forms, charts and references

Keiles Wellness Care Reference Forms for Cleanse/Elimination Diet
http://www.keileswellnesscare.com/referenceform.html

2012 Dirty Dozen Plus and Clean 15
http://www.ewg.org/foodnews/summary/

Foodergies™! Community Forum
http://foodergies.forumcommunity.net

Books/Links to self-assessments that are thorough:

    ଚ୨ Brain Allergies – Dr. William H. Philpott, MD and Dwight K. Kalita, Ph.D.

- The False Fat Diet – Dr. Elson Haas, MD
- Food intolerance questionnaire –
  http://www.thefoodintolerancebible.com
- The UltraSimple Diet – Dr. Mark Hyman, MD
- The Virgin Diet – J.J. Virgin, CNS

Testing facilities for Allergies, Sensitivities and Intolerances

Great Plains Laboratory – IgG with Candida Sensitivity (Dried Blood Spot or Serum blood testing): http://www.greatplainslaboratory.com

Omega Quant Omega-3 Index Test
http://store.drhyman.com/Store/Show/Omega-3-Testing/814/Omega-Quant-HS-Omega-3-Index-Test

DNA (Genetic) Testing For Gluten Sensitivity
http://www.glutenfreesociety.org/product/dna-genetic-testing-for-gluten-sensitivity/

Home Genotyping Kit, Blood Typing Kit – D'Adamo Personalized Nutrition
http://www.4yourtype.com/products.asp?dept=21

GLOSSARY

This is a summary of some of the key items in the book that are referenced. These definitions are more for a cursory explanation – "why it is important" versus a lengthy explanation of the "how and what for."

Vitamins
All natural occurrences of vitamins are found in living things – plants and animals. With a few exceptions our bodies cannot manufacture its own vitamins. These elements need to be sourced from what we eat or by adding supplements to our diets. Vitamins are fat soluble or water soluble. This means how the vitamin is bound – by water or fat – so it can be processed in the body.

Note: it is the nutrient content in the soil in which our foods are grown which directly affects the quality and quantity of vitamins available for us to consume. So if we are adding chemicals to prevent vermin, rot, or genetically engineer our foods – we are inherently changing the capability of the foods to hold their optimum or naturally occurring vitamins. We end up producing nutrient deficient foods.

Vitamin A – A fat soluble vitamin formed from the consumption of retinol (in animal sources) or caretenoids (in plants). This vitamin is essential for our body's normal growth and development along with our visual health. This vitamin is stored in the liver. The vitamin is destabilized by simultaneous exposure to heat and oxygen. Deficiency in Vitamin A results in lowered immunity and negative impact on health of eyes and hair.

Vitamin C – A water soluble vitamin which is absorbed in the small intestine through salt-based processing. It is a key antioxidant necessary for protein collagen formation and helping iron absorption from the plants we eat. It assists in cholesterol conversion to bile acids and creation of Serotonin. Consumption in large quantities can promote diarrhea. Deficiency can result in Scurvy.

Vitamin D – There are two components to Vitamin D. Vitamin D_2 (ergocalciferol) and Vitamin D_3 (cholecalciferol). D2 is derived from plants and yeast. D3 the form of vitamin D we know. When our skin is exposed to direct sunlight it converts the D3 to Calcitriol – the active form of Vitamin D. Calcitriol is necessary for the healthy maintenance of bones. Vitamin D is stored mainly in the liver. Neither D2 nor D3 are active in the body without being processed by liver and kidneys. Calcitriol facilitates absorption of calcium and phosphorus from the intestine. Those two minerals are needed to make bones dense. Vitamin D also enhances immune function and improves muscle strength.

Vitamin E – A fat soluble vitamin which is known in three different forms: Alpha Tocopherol, Beta Tocopherol and Gamma Tocopherol. Vitamin E protects cells (antioxidant) against damage by the by-products of normal cell activity (free-radicals) that participate in chemical reactions. This vitamin is critical to supporting the immune system and our body's metabolic processes.

Vitamin K – A fat soluble vitamin which is heat stable. Comes in two forms: one from plants, Phylloquinone and the other is bacterial, Menaquinone. The Menaquinone is produced by bacteria in the colon and part of immunity. The other is found in highly fermented soy (Natto). Vitamin K also regulates blood coagulation and serum calcium levels.

Thiamine – Also known as B1. This is damaged by exposure to sulfites or alkaki. This water soluble B vitamin is not stored in the body. This vitamin along with all other B Vitamins is used to help synthesize the food we eat into energy and help form blood cells.

Riboflavin – B2 is used to keep the mucous membranes healthy. Also it plays a key role in the metabolism of fats, ketone bodies, carbohydrates, and proteins. It is unstable in light and destroyed by alkali exposure.

Niacin – The B3 vitamin which facilitates glycolysis, fat creation, tissue respiration and cellular energy. This vitamin is hot water and alcohol soluble and can be destroyed by exposure to light, air or alkali.

Vitamin B6 – Is also known as Pyridoxine. This exists in a sensitive balance in our bodies. This water soluble vitamin converts carbohydrates into glucose – the fuel we need at the cellular level. Excess amounts can cause central nervous system impairment.

Folate – This vitamin is also referred to as Folic Acid. Folate is the form that occurs naturally in foods. Folic acid is the manufactured version that is supplemented in our foods. This water soluble vitamin has also been known to reduce homocysteine levels in the blood. Half of the total amount found in the body is stored in the liver.

Pantothenic Acid – One of the B vitamins which helps to converts amino acids and lipids to carbohydrates.

Vitamin B12 – This is one of the key B vitamins called cyanocobalamin. This vitamin is essential for the formation of red blood cells. This vitamin is found in the animals we consume and it is not something we manufacture. Plants have minimal B12 in their systems. Some individual lack the intrinsic factor in their bodies which allows the intestine to extract and process B12. These individuals have to take supplementation to be able to support their red blood cell development.

Betaine – A compound which prevents intracellular osmotic fluid (cell boundary) stress from dehydration. It works with B6, B12 and Folic Acid to reduce the amount of homocysteine in the bloodstream. It is found in the form of Trimethyglicine in plants.

Choline – is a component of phospholipids which are essential for metabolizing carbohydrates and fats. It exists in two forms – free Choline and as Lecithin or Phosphatidylcholine. It also supports protein metabolism, by adding a methyl group to protein during its break down. This is also important for keeping nerve pathways clear and the maintaining the health of the myelin sheaths. It is not technically a vitamin however it is bundled in with the water soluble B vitamins as a critical component to our health.

Minerals and Trace Minerals
Minerals help maintain the delicate water balance in our cells for optimal mental and physical processes.

Calcium – This is the most abundant mineral in the body. It is crucial to the development, maturation and repair of bones. Calcium is critical to the autonomic nervous system control – muscle stimulation, regulation of heart beat, hormones, blood clotting and metabolizing of Vitamin D.

Copper – An important trace mineral found in all body tissues. It is involved in creation of hemoglobin and helps the cell membranes stay healthy. Copper is present in many enzymes which involve the creation or destruction of body tissue. It is also used for the processing of phospholipids, oxidation of Vitamin C to form elastin, and metabolizing proteins.

Fluoride – This mineral is found naturally in sea water, sea vegetables and seafood. Our bones and teeth crystalline structures are fortified by flouride; it combines with the calcium to provide a defense to the native salts in our bones and prevents acid damage.

Iodine – This mineral is processed by our bodies to produce Iodide. This mineral is integral to the proper functioning of the thyroid gland and our hormonal balance.

Iron – This mineral is critical to our bodies as it is the transport mechanism of oxygen from the lungs to the bodily tissues. Iron is the core of the hemoglobin molecule and give our red blood cells that color. Additionally, iron is required for processing of collagen and oxidation of essential fatty acids.

Lithium – A trace mineral which facilitates the neurological balance; must be at a minimum level in the plasma of the bloodstream. Folks on a sodium reduced or free diet may experience toxicity.

Magnesium – This is a workaholic mineral – one with many key functions and can be depleted easily causing deficiencies. Insulin secretion and absorption of calcium, potassium and Vitamin C depend on proper magnesium levels in the body. It also is an activator of the B vitamin complex as well as supporting muscle control/nerve management.

Manganese – Another trace mineral that supports enzymatic reactions in the body, especially relating to maintain of blood sugar and hormone levels.

Phosphorus – This mineral along with calcium are the two key components in bone, teeth and nerve cell formation. It is also the second most abundant mineral in our bodies, next to calcium.

Potassium – This mineral is essential for water balance between cells and the body's fluids as well as maintaining proper heart function. Deficiencies can occur due to diet choices. Some of those signs are muscle cramping, twitching, irregular heart rhythm and kidney failure.

Selenium – This trace mineral has stepped out into the forefront of "wow – did not know how important this is" territory. There are key enzyme reactions in the body that are heavily dependent on proper selenium levels, Selenium acts as an antioxidant and assists with processing of Vitamin D. It is very rare to be deficient with all the variety of foods which have Selenium in them.

Sodium – This mineral is required to manage blood pressure, blood volume and the fluid balance in the body. Sodium is something we get too much of in the Standard American Diet. Many processed and packaged foods contain added Sodium. As a result of the added sodium to our diets, more individuals are getting sodium overload illnesses (dietary hypertension).

Zinc – It is truly the unsung mineral hero. We know it helps fight viruses and shortens cold duration; however it does so much more. Over 300 enzymatic function depend on proper zinc levels in the body. Vegetarians need to consume up to 50% more zinc strong foods to make up for not eating meat.

Key Chemical components

Alkali – Strong base; one of two hydroxides or carbonates, sodium or potassium. The alkali combine with acids to form a salt or with fatty acids to produce soaps.

Cholesterol – A sterol which is synthesized in the liver. It is a part of the bile and one of the main components in gallstones and the plaque in the arteries. It is also required as a pre-cursor to various hormones in the body. It is also found in at least 25% of the brain in the form of myelin.

Dietary Fiber – There are two components of fiber we track in our diets – *Soluble* and *Insoluble*. The *insoluble* adds bulk to bowel movements helping to move the food through the digestive tract, preventing constipation. It also helps clear the toxic by products of the bacteria in the large intestine and alters the pressure in the intestine to prevent diverticulitis. *Soluble* fibers are found in legumes, grains, nuts and seeds. The fiber absorbs the water and turns to gel. This gel slows digestion down.

Fiber in large quantities may hamper the absorption of minerals such as Iron, Zinc, Magnesium, and Calcium in the colon. However plants with high fiber also have high levels of minerals, so there is not as big a concern.

Essential Fatty Acids – A family of fatty acids that are essential to support our good health. Our bodies cannot synthesize them so they need to be consumed from animal and plant fats.

Lectin - A protein in seeds and other parts of certain plants that binds with carbohydrate-protein compounds and carbohydrate-lipid compounds on the surface of animal cells, causing agglutination. Some lectins agglutinate red blood cells in specific blood groups, and others stimulate the production of T lymphocytes (immune response cells). The formal term for a lectin is phytohemagglutinins or hemagglutinins.

Monounsaturated Fat – Increases good cholesterol, lower blood pressure and improves insulin sensitivity when on a reduced carbohydrate diet.

Omega-3 – Also known as alpha linolenic acid or EPA/DHA – necessary along with its related family member of essential fatty acids to support growth and maintenance of cells in our bodies. Key functions performed are managing inflammation, reducing disease promoting molecule in our bodies, improving mood, and behavior. This fatty acid is the one in our diets that tends to be lacking or in lower consumption than Omega-6. There are short chain and long chain versions of this fatty acid – alpha linolenic acid (ALA) is short chain and EPA/DHA are long chain. Plants do not produce long chain – however the body can produce them by converting the ALA to EPA then convert to DHA. Our health is dependent on the proper balance of Omega-3 and Omega-6 in our diets.

Omega-6 – Also known as linoleic acid; it is shown to reduce cholesterol in our bodies when replacing saturated fats, however they trigger inflammatory response and damage blood vessels and can reduce body's effectiveness of processing plant based Omega-3 to EPA/DHA.

Phytosterols – Is a sterol present in vegetable oils or plant based fats. They are known to decrease total and bad cholesterol levels and supports prostate and breast health.

Polyunsaturated Fat – Large amounts of polyunsaturated fatty acids have been shown to increase inflammation, lower good cholesterol in bloodstream and increase release of bile acids; these require Vitamins A, C & E antioxidant properties to counteract their effects.

Saturated Fat – A fat composed of Triglycerides that is made up of saturated fatty acid – the carbon atom in the structure are "saturated" with hydrogen atoms. Saturated fatty acids come in different forms and are in different proportions among food groups. The acids lauric and myristic acids are most commonly found in palm kernel, coconut oil and dairy products. The saturated fatty acids found in meat, eggs, chocolate, and nuts is primarily the triglycerides of palmitic and stearic acids. It is important to watch the consumption of those acids which do not break down easily – like the palmitic and stearic acids. Numerous studies lump both of these types together versus observing the differences in the reactivity in our bodies.

Other Terms

Agglutination – Clumping of cells – antigens, microbes or particles - based on exposure to specific antibodies of an immune response.

Chyme – Partially broken down food and digestive secretions from the stomach and small intestines during the digestion of food consumed.

Flavonoids - The most common group of multi-phenolic compounds in the human diet and are found in all plants. Flavonols, the original bioflavonoids such as Quercetin, are also found all over the plant families, but in lesser quantities. Their variety and the relatively negative impact to health compared to other active chemicals in plants (for instance glycoalkaloids) mean that we may benefit from ingesting significant quantities as part of our diet. Preliminary research shows that flavonoids may be allergen, viral and carcinogenic trigger reducers. Human studies show that flavonoids also have anti-allergic, anti-inflammatory, anti-microbial, anticancer and anti-diarrheal activities.

Food Allergy – Immune response to ingested food which triggers an IgE symptomatic response (see table in Chapter 2). However – there are non IgE allergies to foods as well – and those are more like a food intolerance or sensitivity. Non-IgE allergic reactions by food can also trigger mast cells without being initiated by the IgE immunoglobulin and those have to be dealt with in the same fashion as a traditional IgE allergic response.

Food Intolerance – Intolerance can be from included toxins (poisons), metabolic, pharmacologic or other undefined reactions. A toxin is made by the food itself or by an organism in the food. The toxin can also be something contaminating the food. The interaction with the toxin in our bodies can cause the symptoms of intolerance. Also the body's inability, due to insufficient presence or capability to produce the enzyme needed for digestion, metabolism or removing the toxin/chemical would be described as intolerance.

Food Sensitivity – Abnormal non-immune (not an IgE response) to ingested foods. The component of the broken down food does not mediate a traditional immune response through the mast cells and requires a cumulative build up before generating an immune reaction.

Glycoalkaloids – A family of poisons commonly found in the plant family of *Solanaceae*. A glycoalkaloid is an alkaloid plus sugar combined that could be toxic. One of the most known glycoalkaloid is called *solanine*. It consists of two parts – the sugar *solanose* and the alkaloid *solanidine*. *Solanine* is found in the top most layers of the plants, leaves and stems of the Nightshade family. The largest concentration of solanine is found in the potato tuber just below the skin surface. If you see a green tint to the skin of the potato, it is the *solanine* concentration rising as the potato was exposed to too much sunlight.

The sugar part of the glycoalkaloids is poorly processed by the gastrointestinal tract and can promote gastrointestinal irritation. The alkaloid part of the glycoalkaloid is absorbed into the bloodstream and is believed to be the source of neurological issues. Glycoalkaloids have a bitter taste, and can produce a burning irritation in the back of the mouth and/or side of the tongue when eaten.

Immune Response – The body's response with respect to the presence of foreign antigens so that they become neutralized or eliminated. The body creates immuno-globulin antibodies (IgA, IgE, IgD, IgM, and/or IgG) to prevent injury to the immune system or damage done by foreign invaders.

Oral Allergy Syndrome – Also known as **OAS** - is a type of IgE triggered immune response represented by group of allergic reactions in the mouth in response to eating certain (usually fresh) fruits, nuts and/or vegetables. This syndrome typically develops in adult hay fever sufferers.

Where allergies are concerned, this is probably the most common food-related allergy in adults. OAS is not a separate food allergy, but represents a cross-reactivity between remnants of tree or weed pollen still found in certain fruits and vegetables. As a result, OAS is typically seen in tree and weed allergic patients. It occurs when someone ingests uncooked fruits or vegetables. Unlike other food allergies, in oral allergy syndrome, the reaction is limited to the mouth, lips, tongue and throat. OAS can occur anytime of the year however occurs most frequently the pollen season (spring and fall). Individuals with OAS usually develop symptoms within a few minutes after eating the food.

BIBLIOGRAPHY

Adams, Casey. *Natural Solutions for Food Allergies and Food Intolerances: Scientifically Proven Remedies for Food Sensitivities.* Wilmington, DE: Logical Books, 2011.

Aesoph, Lauri. *How to eat away Arthritis.* Englewood Cliffs, NJ: Prentice Hall, 1996.

Ahern, Shauna James. *Gluten-free girl: how I found the food that loves me back-- & how you can, too.* Hoboken, N.J.: John Wiley & Sons, 2007.

Astor, Stephen. *Hidden Food Allergies.* Garden City Park, N.Y.: Avery Pub. Group, 1988.

Bohager, Tom. *Everything you need to know about enzymes: a simple guide to using enzymes to treat everything from digestive problems and allergies to migraines and arthritis.* Austin, TX: Greenleaf Book Group Press, 2008.

Bowden, Jonny. *The 150 Healthiest Foods on Earth: The Surprising, Unbiased Truth About What You Should Eat and Why.* Gloucester, MA: Fair Winds Press, 2007.

Bower, Sylvia Llewelyn, Sharrett, Mary Kay and Plogsted, Steve. *Celiac disease: a guide to living with gluten intolerance.* New York, N.Y.: Demos, 2006.

Braly, James, Holdford, Patrick. *Hidden Food Allergies: The essential guide to uncovering hidden food allergies – and achieving permanent relief.* Laguna Beach, CA: Basic Health Publications Inc., 2005.

Brostoff, Jonathan and Gamlin, Linda. *Food allergies and food intolerance: the complete guide to their identification and treatment.* Rochester, VT. : Healing Arts Press, 2000.

Brynie, Faith Hickman. *101 Questions about your Immune System: You felt defenseless to answer...until now.* Brookfield, CT.: Twenty-First Century Books, 2000.

Carper, Jean. *Food – Your Miracle Medicine.* New York: HarperCollins Publishers, 1993.

Carper, Jean. *The Food Pharmacy.* New York: Bantam Books, 1988.

Case, Shelley. *Gluten-free diet: a comprehensive resource.* Regina, AB: Case Nutrition, Consulting, 2001.

Cass, Hyla. *Supplement your prescription: what your doctor doesn't know about nutrition.* Laguna Beach, CA: Basic Health Pub, 2007.

Childers, Norman Franklin and Russo, Gerard M. *Nightshades and Health.* Somerville, NJ: Somerset Press Inc., 1977.

Childers, Norman F. *Arthritis – The Diet That Stops It: The Nightshades, Ill health, Aging and Shorter Life (6th Edition).* Gainsville, FL: Dr. Norman F Childers Publications, 1999.

Crook, William G. *Tracking Down Hidden Food Allergy (6th Printing).* Jackson, TN. Professional Books: 1985.

Crook, William G. and Jones, Marjorie Hunt. *The Yeast Connection Cookbook: A guide to good nutrition and better health.* Jackson, TN, Professional Books: 2005.

Cutler, Ellen. *The Food Allergy Cure (1st Ed).* New York, NY: Three Rivers Press, 2003.

D'Adamo, Peter and Whitney, Catherine. *Cook right 4 your type: the practical kitchen companion to eat right 4 your type, including more than 200 original recipes, as well as individualized 30-day meal plans for staying healthy, living longer, and achieving your ideal weight.* New York, NY: G.P. Putnam's Sons, 1998.

D'Adamo, Peter and Whitney, Catherine. *Arthritis: fight it with the blood type diet.* New York, NY: Berkeley Publishing Group, 2004.

Daniluk, Julie. *Meals that heal inflammation: Embrace healthy living and eliminate pain, one meal at a time.* Carlsbad, CA. Hay House, 2011.

Dennis, Melinda and Leffler, Daniel A. *Real life with celiac disease: troubleshooting and thriving gluten free.* Bethesda, MD: AGA Press, 2010.

Desrochers, Pierre and Shimizu, Hiroko. *The locavore's dilemma: in praise of the 10,000-mile diet.* New York: Public Affairs, 2012.

Deville, Nancy. *Death by supermarket: the fattening, dumbing down, and poisoning of America.* Austin, Tex.: Greenleaf Book Group Press, 2011.

Diamond, Elizabeth Ann. *Nutritional Medicine A-Z of Disease & Illness.* Amazon Kindle.com/com.uk. : 2011.

Fitzgerald, Randall. *The Hundred-Year Lie: how food and medicine are destroying your health.* New York, NY: Dutton, 2006.

Freund, Lee H. and Rejaunier, Jeanne. *Complete idiot's guide to food allergies.* Indianapolis, IN: Alpha, 2003.

Fowler, Michael. *Nightshade Free, Pain Free!* Stockton, CA: Grass Fire Media: 2007.

Gaby, Alan R. *Nutritional Medicine.* Concord, NH: Fritz Perlberg Publishing, 2011.

Gilbère, Gloria. *Designing Health, Naturally: Volume 1 - Pain/inflammation matters.* Lancaster, OH: Lucky Press, 2005.

Gordon, Sherri Mabry. *Peanut butter, milk, and other deadly threats: what you should know about food allergies.* Berkeley Heights, NJ: Enslow Publishers, 2006.

Graci, Sam. *The Food Connection: the right food at the right time.* Mississauga, Ontario: John Wiley & Sons, Canada, Ltd., 2006

Green, Peter H. R. and Jones, Rory. *Celiac disease: a hidden epidemic.* New York: William Morrow, 2010.

Guyol, Gracelyn. *Healing depression & bipolar disorder without drugs: inspiring stories of restoring mental health through natural therapies.* New York: Walker & Company, 2006.

Haas, Elson M. and Levin, Buck. *Staying Healthy with Nutrition: The Complete Guide to Diet and Nutritional Medicine.* Berkeley, CA: Celestial Arts, 2006.

Haas, Elson M. and Stauth, Cameron. *The False Fat Diet – The Revolutionary 21-Day Program for Losing the Weight You Think is Fat.* New York: Ballantine Books, 2001.

Haas, Elson M. and Chase, Daniella. *The New Detox Diet: The Complete Guide for Lifelong Vitality With Recipes, Menus, and Detox Plans (2nd Edition).* Berkeley, CA: Celestial Arts, 2004.

Haynes, Antony J. and Savill, Antoinette. *The Food Intolerance Bible: A Nutritionist's Plan to Beat Food Cravings, Fatigue, Mood Swings, Bloating, Headaches, IBS and Deal with Food Allergies.* London, UK: HarperCollins, 2008 (Kindle Edition)

Hausman, Patricia and Hurley, Judith Benn. *The Healing Foods – The Ultimate Authority on the Curative Power of Nutrition.* Emmaus, PA: Rodale Press, 1989.

Heiser, Charles Bixler. *Nightshades; the paradoxical plants.* San Francisco, CA: W. H. Freeman, 1969.

Hicks, J. Morris and Hicks, J. Stanfield. *Healthy eating, healthy world: unleashing the power of plant-based nutrition.* Dallas, TX: BenBella Books, 2011.

Jensen, Bernard. *Dr. Jensen's Guide to Better Bowel Care: A Complete Program for tissue cleansing through bowel management.* New York, NY: Avery/Penguin Putnam: 1999.

Jensen, Bernard. *Foods that Heal: a guide to understanding and using the healing powers of natural foods.* New York, NY: Avery/Penguin Putnam: 1993.

Joneja, Janice M. Vickerstaff. *Dealing with food allergies: a practical guide to detecting culprit foods and eating a healthy, enjoyable diet.* Boulder, Colo.: Bull Pub., 2003.

Kamhi, Ellen and Zampieron, Eugene R. *Alternative medicine definitive guide to arthritis: reverse underlying causes of arthritis with clinically proven alternative therapies (2nd Edition).* Berkley, CA: Celestial Arts, 2006

Kirchfeld, Friedhelm and Boyle, Wade. *Nature Doctors: Pioneers in Naturopathic Medicine.* Portland, Oregon: NCNM Press, 1994

Kirschmann, John D. and Nutrition Search, Inc. *Nutrition Almanac (6th Edition).* New York: McGraw-Hill, 2007.

Li, Thomas S.C. *Vegetables and Fruits – Nutritional and Therapeutic Values.* New York: CRC Press (Taylor & Francis Group), 2008.

Lieberman, Shari and Segall, Linda. *The gluten connection: how gluten sensitivity may be sabotaging your health-- and what you can do to take control now.* New York, NY: Rodale, 2007.

Magee, Elaine. *Food Synergy: Unleash Hundreds of Powerful Healing Food Combinations to Fight Disease and Live Well.* New York: Rodale. 2007.

Martin, Raquel and Romano, Karen J. *Preventing and Reversing Arthritis Naturally: The Untold Story.* Rochester, VT: Healing Arts Press, 2000.

Melina, Vesanto, Stepaniak, Jo and Aronson, Dina. *Food allergy survival guide: surviving and thriving with food allergies and sensitivities.* Summertown, Tenn.: Healthy Living Publications, 2004.

Meyerowitz, Steve. *Food combining and digestion: 101 ways to improve digestion.* Great Barrington, MA: Sproutman Publications, 2002

Mindell, Earl and Mundis, Hester. *Unsafe at any meal: how to avoid hidden toxins in your food.* Chicago: Contemporary Books, 2002.

Niazian, Bethany. *Food Allergies Beyond the Top 8: A Substitution Guide.* Amazon Digital Services, Inc. 2012 (Kindle Edition).

Ochel, Evita. *Healing & Prevention Through Nutrition: Natural and holistic approach for How to Eat, What to Eat and Why for optimal health and wellness.*

Amazon Createspace, 2011 (Kindle Edition)

Philpott, William H and Kalita, Dwight K. *Brain Allergies: The Psychonutrient and Magnetic Connections (2nd Edition)*. Los Angeles: Keats Publishing, 2000.

Pickering, Wayne. *Food Combining for Health and Longevity* (Kindle Edition) Dayton Beach, FL: The Center for Nutrition, 2011

Pickell, Melissa. *Marvelous meatless meals: everyday recipes those are free of gluten, dairy, and refined sugar*. Flemington, N.J.: New You Nutrition, 2008.

Rachlitz, Steven. *Allergies and Candida with the Physicists Rapid Solution. (4th Ed.)* Sedona, AZ. Human Ecology Balancing Science: 2000.

Rapaport, Howard G and Linde, Shirley Motter. *The Complete Allergy Guide*. New York: Simon and Schuster, 1970.

Reed, Penny Kendall and Reed, Stephen. *Healing Arthritis: Dietary Treatment for Arthritis*. Ontario, QC: CCNM Press, 2004.

Rivera, Rudy and Deutsch, Roger D. *Your Hidden Food Allergies are Making You Fat*. Rocklin, Calif.: Prima Health, 1998.

Ross, Julia. *The Diet Cure: The 8-Step Program to Rebalance Your Body Chemistry and End Food Cravings, Weight Problems, and Mood Swings-Now*. New York, NY: Viking Penguin, 1999.

Shepard, Jules E. Dowler. *The first year: celiac disease and living gluten-free: an essential guide for the newly diagnosed*. Cambridge, MA: Da Capo Press, 2008.

Shils, Maurice E (Senior Editor) and Shike, Moshe, et al (Associate Editors). *Modern Nutrition in health and disease (10th Edition)*. Baltimore, MD: Lippincott Williams & Wilkins, 2006.

Skypala, Isabel and Venter, Carina (Editors). *Food Hypersensitivity: Diagnosing and Managing Food Allergies and Intolerance*. West Sussex, UK: Wiley-Blackwell Publishing Ltd., 2009

Smith, Melissa Diane. *Going against the grain: how reducing and avoiding grains can revitalize your health.* Chicago, IL: Contemporary Books, 2002.

Spicer, Elizabeth F. *Ask your body: relieve your food allergies instantly and naturally with muscle testing.* Blue Hill, Maine: Medicine Bear Pub., 1998.

Tessmer, Kimberly A. *Tell me what to eat if I have celiac disease: nutrition you can live with.* Franklin Lakes, NJ: New Page Books, 2009.

Tessmer, Kimberly A. *Gluten-free for a healthy life: nutritional advice and recipes for those suffering from celiac disease and other gluten-related disorders.* Franklin Lakes, NJ: New Page Books, 2003

Thomson, Peter. *Complete Food Combining – All you need to know about the Hay Diet.* Kindle Edition 2011.

Venes, Donald (Editor). *Taber's Cyclopedic Medical Dictionary (20th Edition).* Philadelphia, PA: F. A. Davis Company: 2005.

Walsh, William E. *Food allergies: the complete guide to understanding and relieving your food allergies.* New York: J. Wiley, 2000.

Wangen, Stephen. *Healthier without Wheat: A New Understanding of Wheat Allergies, Celiac Disease and Non-celiac Gluten Intolerance.* Seattle, WA: Innate Health Publishing, 2009.

Weil, Andrew. *Natural Health, Natural Medicine: A comprehensive manual for wellness and self-care.* Boston: Houghton Mifflin Company, 1990

ONLINE REFERENCES

Bio Individuality and Human Genome
ABO Blood Types: http://anthro.palomar.edu/blood/ABO_system.htm

Sub Groups of A: D'Adamo, Peter J. 2009 from online
dadamonutrition.com

ABO Blood Group Polymorphism: D'Adamo, Peter J. 2009 from online
dadamonutrition.com

Mind Guide to Food and Mood
http://www.mind.org.uk/help/medical_and_alternative_care/food_and_m
ood-the_mind_guru.

IgG Food Allergies.pdf from the Great Plains Laboratory
www.greatplainslaboratory.com

The Healing Crisis from www.falconblanco.com/health/crisis.htm

http://www.agedefyingbody.com/regenerationschedule.html

Ancient cycle of cellular regeneration – by Charlotte J. Carreira, Simplexity
Simple Solutions: Vol 8, Issue 4 www.wholefoodwellness.net

Food Combining/Cross reactivity/Diet implications
Incompatible Food Combinations via Ayurvedic medicine: Lad, Dr. Vasant
1994 from http://www.healthy.net/scr/article.aspx?397

Puristat Digestive Wellness Center
http://www.puristat.com/foodcombiningchart_2.aspx

ABCompany.com Food Combinations & Choices: Food Combining
Chart2.pub (as PDF)

García, BE et al, **Cross-reactivity Syndromes in Food Allergy.** J Investig Allergol Clin Immunol 2011; Vol. 21(3): 162-170 © 2011 Esmon Publicidad (PDF)

Lewey, Scot. EZineArticles: **Food Allergies, Intolerance and Adverse Reactions Associated With Specific Pollens**
http://ezinearticles.com/?Food-Allergies,-Intolerance-and-Adverse-Reactions-Associated-With-Specific-Pollens&id=306107

Food Combining Chart – A Naturopathic perspective 2012-08-04
http://www.ndhealthfacts.org/Food_Combining_chart.html

Getting Started with Healthy Eating – Elimination Diet
http://www.getting-started-with-healthy-eating.com/elimination-diet.html

Food Family Lists
Food Allergy Gourmet – Botanical Food Families
http://www.foodallergygourmey.com/Food%20Allergy/Food%20Families.htm

AAIA: Food Groups http://www.aaia.ca/en/food_groups.htm

The Alternative Doctor – Allergy Section – FOOD ALLERGY: Food Families? http://www.alternative-doctor.com/allergies/foodfamilies.html

Food Intolerances in Fatigue Syndromes
http://www.thenaturalrecoveryplan.com/food-intolerances.html

Fairfield County Allergy, Asthma & Immunology Associates, P.C. Food Family List.PDF

Getting Started with Healthy Eating – Food Families
http://www.getting-started-with-healthy-eating.com/food-families.html

Innvista – Food Families
http://www.innvista.com/foods/food-families/

Nutritional Information
Eat Right For Your Type: TypeBase 4 BTD Food Values from
http://www.dadamo.com/typebase4/typeindexer.htm

CureZone Food lists: http://curezone.com/ER4YT

Nutrition Data: http://nutritiondata.self.com

Dr. Decuypere's Nutrient Charts - http://www.health-alternatives.com/

About Nuts: Nuts in a healthy lifestyle –
http://www.aboutnuts.com/en/enzyklopaedie

University of Maryland Medical Center – Online Reference:
Complementary Medicine
http://www.umm.edu/altmed/articles/brewers-Yeast-000288.htm

Innvista references on individual plants
http://www.innvista.com/foods/food-families/
Subdocuments as needed

Botanical Online
http://www.botanical-online.com/english/
Subdocuments as needed

The World's Healthiest Foods http://www.whfoods.com

References
Cassaro, Richard. The Ancient "Doctrine of Signatures" Suppressed By The Establishment. Blog Post. *December 1st, 2011*
http://www.richardcassaro.com/the-ancient-doctrine-of-signatures-suppressed-by-the-elite

J.Crows: The Household Physician – Doctrine of Signatures
http://www.jcrows.com/signatures.html

Vasquez, Alex et al. **THE CLINICAL IMPORTANCE OF VITAMIN**

D (CHOLECALCIFEROL): A PARADIGM SHIFT WITH IMPLICATIONS FOR ALL HEALTHCARE PROVIDERS. ALTERNATIVE THERAPIES, SEPT/OCT 2004, VOL. 10, NO. 5. http://optimalhealthresearch.com/reprints/vasquez-manso-cannell-vitamindmonograph-athm.pdf

Nightshades – Weston A Price Foundation: Smith, Garrett. Spring 2010 – Updated April 2 2012. Wise Traditions in Food, Farming and the Healing Arts.

Marshall Protocol Study Site – Calcitriol content in foods. April 10, 2010. http://www.marshallprotocol.com/forum11/13722.html

Health Canada – Glycoalkaloids in Foods http://www.hc-sc.gc.ca/fn-an/pubs/securit/2010-glycoalkaloids-glycoalcaloides/index-eng.php

Canadian Food Inspection Agency – Natural Toxins in Fresh Fruits and Vegetables. http://www.inspection.gc.ca/food/consumer-centre/food-safety-tips/specific-products-and-risks/natural-toxins/eng/1332276569292/1332276685336

Nightshade Foods – Organic Foodie. Sims, Craig (downloaded 8/7/2012) http://www.organicfoodee.com/inspiration/craig/nightshadefoods/

Solanine Toxicity Syndrome (downloaded 8/7/2012) http://www.michaellebowitzdc.com/html/Solanine.html

Friedman, M. Analysis of biologically active compounds in Potatoes (Solanum tuberosum), Tomatoes (Lycopersicon esculentum), and jimson weed (Datura stramonium) seeds. J. Chromatogr. A. 2004 Oct 29; 1054 (1-2): 143-55. http://ncbi.nlm.nih.gov/pubmed/15553139

Friedman, Mendel. Potato Glycoalkaloids and Metabolites: Roles in the Plant and in the Diet. J. Agric. Food Chem., 2006, 54 (23) pp.8655 – 8681 (Web Publication date October 20, 2006)

Milner, Sinead, et al. **Bioactivities of Glycoalkaloids and their Aglycones from *Solanum* Species**. J. Agric. Food Chem., 2011, 59 (8) pp.3454 – 3484 (Web Publication date March 14, 2011)

Living with Phytic Acid – Weston A Price Foundation: Nagel, Ramiel. Spring 2010 (26 March 2010); updated 02 April 2012.

Tarleton, Sherry and DiBaise, John K., **Low-Residue Diet in Diverticular Disease: Putting an End to a Myth.** *Nut Clin Pract* 2011 26: 137 (downloaded from Sage Publications online http://ncp.sagepub.com/content/26/2/137

Molyneux, Russell J., Mahoney, Noreen, Kim, Jong H., Campbell, Bruce C. **Mycotoxins in edible Tree nuts**. International Journal of Food Microbiology 119 (2007) 72–78. PDF from sciencedirect.com

Risky Foods from online betterhealthblog.com Oct 1 2012

Kessman, Scott. **Health benefits of eating Venison**. Nov 16, 2010. http://voices.yahoo.com/health-benefits-venison-7170060.html

The World's Healthiest Foods – Venison in depth (and other references) http://www.whfoods.com/genpage.php?tname=nutrientprofile&dbid=6

Food Allergies and Intolerances Resource List for Consumers December 2010 http://www.nal.usda.gov/fnic/pubs/bibs/allergy.pdf

IgE versus Non IgE Reactions – Ask the Doc:
What's the difference between food allergy and food intolerance?
http://apfed.org/drupal/drupal/sites/default/files/files/IgE%20vs%20nonIgE%20reactions.pdf

What is Celiac Disease? - Celiac Disease and Systemic Enzymes – written 17 January 2011 http://www.inflammation-systemicenzymes.com/celiac-disease-.html?start=1

Dr. Peter Osborne – Gluten Free Society: May 23, 2011
http://www.glutenfreesociety.org/gluten-free-society-blog/doctor-denial-why-most-doctors-ignore-gluten-sensitivity/

Dr. Peter Osborne – Gluten Free Society: February 22, 2012
http://www.glutenfreesociety.org/gluten-free-society-blog/why-are-some-doctors-scarred-of-gluten-sensitivity/

Lewey, Scot. EZineArticles: **Genetics of Food Allergy and Intolerance**.
http://ezinearticles.com/?Genetics-of-Food-Allergy-and-Intolerance&id=301254

Agri Analysis, Inc. **Testing Cereal Grains for Prolamin**.
www.agrianalysis.com – Testing for Prolamin.PDF

"Facts about Hemp" (http://www.ecofibre.com.au/facts.html). Ecofibre Industries. http://www.ecofibre.com.au/facts.html.

"Wilde Country Rancho Hemp Products"
(http://www.wcranchoHemp.com/info.php). WcranchoHemp.com.
http://www.wcranchoHemp.com/info.php.

http://www.drbronner.com/pdf/Hempnutrition.pdf
http://www.getting-started-with-healthy-eating.com/lists-of-nuts.html

Callaway JC (2004). **Hemp seed as a nutritional resource: an overview**. Euphytica 140:65-72.

(Hemp Seeds are full of Health) 9/14/2010 Christen Peattie, HHP
http://www.naturalnews.com/029729_Hemp_seeds_health.html

Rice with human proteins takes root in Kansas by Emma Marris May 17, 2007 – Nature News
http://www.bioedonline.org/news/news.cfm?art=3335

Huang, Q et al. **Anticancer properties of anthraquinones from Rhubarb**. Med Res Rev 2007 September 27; 27(5) pp 609-630.

http://www.ncbi.nlm.nih.gov/pubmed/17022020

Little-White, Heather (Contributor) **Sorrel, so divine!** The Jamaica Gleaner (online) http://jamaica-gleaner.com/gleaner/20091212/features/features8.html

Tropical Plant Database entry for: Maca- Lepidium meyenii http://www.rain-tree.com/maca.htm

Adel, Shirin and Prakash, Jamuna. **The Chemical Composition and Antioxidant Properties of ginger root (Zingiber officinale).** Journal of Medicinal Plants Research Vol. 4(24), pp. 2674-2679. 18 December 2010 http://www.academicjournals.org/JMPR

Whitney, Martha. Dr. Christopher's Herbal Legacy – Ginger. http://www.herballegacy.com/Whitney_Chemical.html http://www.herballegacy.com/Whitney_Medicinal.html

Medline Plus for definitions http://www.nlm.nih.gov/medlineplus/ency/

Merck Manual Home Heath Handbook http://www.merckmanuals.com/home/print/disorders_of_nutrition/Vitamins/

Medline Plus - Soluble vs Insoluble Fiber http://www.nlm.nih.gov/medlineplus/ency/article/002136.htm

ND Health Facts http://www.ndhealthfacts.org/wiki/Main_Page

Schiffner R, Przybilla B, Burgdorff T, Landthaler M, Stolz W (October 2001). **Anaphylaxis to buckwheat.** *Allergy* **56** (10): 1020–1. http://www.ncbi.nlm.nih.gov/pubmed/11576091

Pine nuts nutrition facts and health benefits http://www.nutrition-and-you.com/pine_nuts.html

Aronson, Dina and Kimmel, Dina. **Ancient Foods which are nutritional gems today.** NAVS _ North American Vegetarian Societynuts and seeds.pdf 12/23/2012. navs@telenet.net

Dr. Decuypere's Nutrient Charts - http://www.health-alternatives.com/

Spark People – Calories in Lifeway Lowfat Kefir
http://www.sparkpeople.com/calories-in.asp?food=Kefir

Linus Pauling Institute at Oregon State University – Phytosterols
http://lpi.oregonstate.edu/infocenter/phytochemicals/sterols

CompositDB – A brief overview of Compositae, Lettuce and Sunflower
http://compositdb.ucdavis.edu/compositae_overview.php

Björkhem, Ingemar and Meaney, Steve. **Brain Cholesterol: Long Secret Life Behind a Barrier.** Arteriosclerosis, Thrombosis, and Vascular Biology. **2004;** 24: **806-815** *Published online before print February 5, 2004,* **doi: 10.1161/01.ATV.0000120374.59826.1b**
http://atvb.ahajournals.org/content/24/5/806.full.pdf+html

Reducing Pain and Inflammation Naturally. Part II: New Insights into Fatty Acid Supplementation and Its Effect on Eicosanoid Production and Genetic Expression by Alex Vasquez, D.C., and N.D. Published January 2005 in *Nutritional Perspectives: Journal of the Council on Nutrition of the American Chiropractic Association*
http://optimalhealthresearch.com/reprints/series/vasquez_part2_2005_fat tyacidmonograph.pdf

Enman, Josefine. **Production and Quantification of Eritadenine, Cholesterol Reducing Compound in Shiitake *(Lentinus edodes)* -** May 2007. http://epubl.ltu.se/1402-1757/2007/26/LTU-LIC-0726-SE.pdf

Koyyalamudi SR, Jeong SC, Song CH, Cho KY, Pang G (April 2009). **Vitamin D2 formation and bioavailability from Agaricus bisporus button Mushrooms treated with ultraviolet irradiation.** J Agric Food Chem 57 (8): 3351–5. http://www.ncbi.nlm.nih.gov/pubmed/19281276

Lin, David C. **Probiotics As Functional Foods.** *Nutr Clin Pract* 2003 18:

497 http://ncp.sagepub.com/content/18/6/497

Powerful Health Benefits of the Pomegranate – Dr.Furhman
http://www.drfuhrman.com/library/article19.aspx

Foods High In Lithium | LIVESTRONG.COM Jul 27, 2011 | By
JacobS: http://www.livestrong.com/article/502977-foods-high-in-lithium/?utm_source=popslideshow

What Foods Contain Lithium? | LIVESTRONG.COM Aug 18, 2011 |
By Suzanne Allen
http://www.livestrong.com/article/519437-what-foods-contain-lithium/

Schrauzer, G.N. Journal of the American College of Nutrition – **Lithium:
Occurrence, Dietary Intakes, Nutritional Essentiality**. February 2002
http://www.jacn.org/content/21/1/14.full

Wilson, Lawrence MD. Lithum. Center for Development. January 2012.
http://drlwilson.com/ARTICLES/LITHIUM.htm

Lithium-Rich Foods |Why You Need Lithium |Comprehensive Review
http://www.collectivewizdom.com/Lithium-LithiumRichFoods.html

Essence-of-Life: Health Topics - Lithium
http://www.essense-of-life.com/product_A-212/.htm

Zinc: Essential for human health. International Zinc Association
http://www.zinc.org/info/zinc_essential_for_human_health

Discovery Fit & Health - What are some common fish allergy symptoms?
http://health.howstuffworks.com/diseases-conditions/allergies/food-allergy/shellfish/common-fish-allergy-symptoms.htm

Composition of Kiwi Fruit
http://www.food-allergens.de/symposium-vol1(1)/data/kiwi/kiwi-composition.htm

Okra facts -http://foodsthatheal.blogspot.com/2007/02/okra.html

Correspondence: **Safety of Carageenan in Foods** – by Phil Carthew. Unilever Safety and Environmental. VOLUME 110 | NUMBER 4 | April 2002, Pg 176. Environmental Health Perspectives. http://www.ncbi.nlm.nih.gov/pmc/articles/PMC1240817/pdf/ehp0110-a0176b.pdf

Correspondence: **Carrageenan in Foods: Response** – by Joanne Tobacman. University of Iowa Health Care. VOLUME 110 | NUMBER 4 | April 2002, Pg 176-177. Environmental Health Perspectives. http://www.ncbi.nlm.nih.gov/pmc/articles/PMC1240817/pdf/ehp0110-a0176b.pdf

Benard, Claudine et al. **Degraded Carrageenan Causing Colitis in Rats Induces TNF Secretion and ICAM-1 Upregulation in Monocytes through NF-kB Activation.** www.plosone.org. January 2010 | Volume 5 | Issue 1 | e8666

Talero Elena, et al. **Anti-Inflammatory Effects of Adrenomedullin on Acute Lung Injury Induced by Carrageenan in Mice.** Hindawi Publishing Corporation: Mediators of Inflammation. Volume 2012, Article ID 717851, 13 pages. doi:10.1155/2012/717851

INDEX

A

Absinthe 42
aches 13, 94-5
acidic 154-5
acids, stearic 109, 111, 174
Adzuki Bean 83
Aflatoxin 86-7, 99, 107
agglutination 84, 101, 172, 174
ALA see alpha linolenic acid
albumin, key proteins 108
alkali 169, 172
alkaloids 26, 35, 135, 138, 175
allergic ii, 8, 34, 57, 76, 96, 117, 134, 164
allergic reactions 110, 155, 175
allergies 7-9, 13, 16-17, 26, 30, 35, 55, 64, 72-3, 81, 89, 97, 115, 122, 157, 166, 175
   milk protein 64
allergy elimination diet 96
almonds 26, 45, 96-7, 106-7, 117, 164
Aloe/Aloe Tea/Aloe Juice 163
alpha linolenic acid (ALA) 108, 173
Alpha Tocopherol 98, 100, 103-4, 106, 168
amaranth 39, 56, 58, 126
amygdalin 97, 151-2
analgesic 91, 143, 158-9
animal proteins 32, 57, 61, 69, 75-6, 80-2, 96, 160, 164
   most consumed 68
   optimal 75
Animal Proteins & Dairy 61, 75-6
anthocyanins 53, 130, 136, 141, 144, 148-9
anthraquinones 149-50
anti-inflammatory 91, 98, 105-6, 113, 121, 134, 149, 156, 159, 174
antibacterial 91, 98, 100, 112, 128, 133-5, 139, 142, 152, 156, 159

antibiotics 65, 69, 121, 128
antibodies 8-10, 174
anticancer 91, 112, 128, 133, 139, 158, 174
anticancer properties 131, 135, 149, 152
anticoagulant 127-8, 139, 157-9
antigens 10-11, 174
antioxidant properties 53, 91, 102-3, 106, 114, 121, 126, 128, 130-1, 133-4, 136, 138-9, 141-2,149, 152-4, 156, 158, 168, 171, 173
   strong 127, 129
apples 25-6, 35, 45, 76, 150-2, 161, 164
apricot 45, 106, 150-1, 160
arachidonic acid 63-4, 75
arthritis 3-4, 6, 26, 31, 89
artichokes 137-8, 163
Asparagus 40, 130-1
avocado 44, 142-3, 162

B

B-Vitamin Complex 119
B Vitamins 168-9, 171
Bacon 36, 67-8
bacteria 72, 75, 118, 121, 168, 172
bacterium 69
Baker's Yeast 46, 118-19, 121, 124
balance 5, 33, 109, 121-2, 130, 136, 139, 153
   excellent 65-6
   unhealthy 109
   water/sodium 147-8
banana 44, 57, 146-7, 160-2
Barley 38, 49, 51, 58
Barracuda 37, 79
Bass 37, 79-80
beans 39, 82, 84, 86, 153
beef 29, 36, 64-6, 69, 76, 78-9, 81,

122
Beet Juice 163
beets 38, 56, 126-7
Bell Pepper 7, 89-91
Belladonna 45, 88
Beta-carotene 91, 146
Betaine 56, 68, 70, 102-4, 120, 126-7, 147, 169
bioflavonoids 129, 131, 154, 157, 174
Black Bean 39, 82-3, 86
black trumpet 118, 122-4
Blood Type Impacts 58, 77, 85, 93, 116, 123, 161
blueberries 43, 141-2, 162
Bluegill Bass 79
bowel movements 17, 22, 172
bowels 22-3, 122
Bran 58
Brazil Nut 44, 103, 116
breads 18, 49, 59, 64, 118
broccoli 29, 41, 107, 132, 163-4
Bromelain 134
buckwheat 39, 48, 55, 58-9, 149
buckwheat family members 149
Buckwheat/Kasha 58-9
Bulgur 38, 49-50, 58
Butter 35, 62-3, 116

C

Cabbage 41, 132, 163
caffeine 20, 33, 153
Calcitriol 7, 91-2, 168
calcium 56, 62, 106, 108, 112-13, 126, 132, 137-8, 144, 149, 156, 170-2
calcium deposits 4
Campylobacter 69
cancers 98, 150
Cantaloupe 42, 138-9, 160
Capsicum Peppers 90-1
Carambola 44, 162
Carob 39, 82, 84
Carrageenan 64
carrots 46, 155-6, 163
cashews 29, 40, 98-9, 128-9

catechins 100, 106-7, 145-6, 151
Catfish 37, 70-1, 79
Cauliflower 41, 132-3, 163
Caviar 79-80
Cayenne Pepper 93
celeriac 46, 155-6
celery 46, 155-6
celiac 19, 48-9
celiac disease 4, 6, 12, 54
cells 15, 75, 101, 128, 156, 168, 170-1, 173-4
    mast 10, 174-5
    red blood 169-70, 172
chard 38, 56, 126-7
charts 51-2, 165
cheeses 35, 62
chemical instructions 25
cherry 45, 106, 150-1, 160, 162
chestnuts 43, 101, 116
chew 7, 75, 139
chia seeds 44, 112-13
chicken 12, 36, 63, 68-69, 76, 78
    pastured 69
Chickpeas 39, 82-4
Chicory 42, 137, 163
chocolate 44, 76, 144-5, 161, 174
choices, prior diet/lifestyle 31
cholesterol 63, 65, 68-9, 71, 73, 98-9, 101, 107, 110-11, 114, 136, 140, 152, 172-3
cholesterol diet, low 53
Choline 56, 68, 70, 72, 103-4, 106, 120, 126-7, 129, 131-2, 134, 138, 143, 148-9, 169
cinnamon 44, 142-3
clams 38, 73-4, 79, 81
cleanse/fast 22
cleanses 13-14, 16, 18, 20-2, 35
cocoa 44, 144-5
coconut 40, 99, 103, 117, 129
Cod 37, 70, 80
coffee 20, 33, 45, 152-3, 161
Cola 161
Cola Nut 44, 144
colon 17, 22-3, 52-3, 107, 113, 121,

139, 168, 172
Community Forum   164-5
Conch   38, 79
constipation   12, 22-3, 150
contamination   52-3
contraceptive   145
Copper   50, 55-6, 68, 72, 74, 83, 100, 102-6, 109-11, 113, 131, 143-4, 170
corn   18, 38, 48-51, 53-4, 57, 71, 75, 161
Couscous   58
cow   75, 77-8
Crab   38, 72-3, 79
Cracked Wheat   58
cranberries   43, 141-2
Cravings   33-4
Croaker   37
Crocodiles   36
crustaceans   9, 29, 38, 72, 74, 97
Cucumber   42, 138-9, 163
currants   46, 157, 160

D

dairy   5, 9, 13, 15, 18, 35, 52, 61, 63-4, 75-8, 80-1, 92, 114, 145, 160, 173
dairy group members   80
Dandelion   42, 137, 163
Deadly Nightshade   88
Deer   36, 66
deficiencies   4, 9, 14, 34, 167-8, 171
detritus   73, 81
diet   1-2, 4, 16, 21-9, 54-5, 61-2, 68-9, 71-2, 88-9, 96-9, 103-7, 125-6, 128-32, 134-8, 140-3, 145-9, 151-2, 154-5, 157-8, 171-4
   current   17, 33
   elimination   97
   elimination/challenge   19
   free   171
   human   174
   normal   65
   plant-based   64
   proper   71
   reduced   96
   rotation   86
   snacking   89
diet choices   14, 27, 171
diet elimination   60
diet lifestyle programs   25
dietary elimination   35
   performed   12
dietary elimination challenge-response diet   4
dietary evaluations   7
dietary hypertension   171
dietary interactions, observing   30
digestive health   20, 53
   supporting   56
digestive system   7, 22-3, 159
Diosgenin   140
Dirty Dozen   159, 165
diuretic   131, 134, 140, 150, 153
   properties   144-5
Doctrine of Signatures   84, 91, 103, 146, 155-6, 159
DPPIV   52
Duck   36, 68, 78
Dust Mite Allergy   160-1

E

ears   121
eczema   29, 60
Edestin   108
Eel   38, 79
EFA see essential fatty acids
Egg Yolk   62-3
eggplant   45, 89-93
eggs   12, 18, 36, 62-4, 66, 75-6, 81, 112-13, 161, 174
Eicosanoids   114
elimination diet style exercise   18
endive   42, 137
enzymes   8, 35, 54, 57, 75-6, 102, 126, 146, 152, 170, 175
EPA/DHA   173
Erepsine   139
Ergothioneine   121
Eritadenine   121

Escarole   42, 137, 163
essential fatty acids (EFA)   53, 56, 69,
103-4, 106, 108-9, 111, 120, 135, 148,
152, 170, 172-3

F

fasts   2, 20-1
fatty acids   172-3
  saturated   173-4
fauna   14, 28-9, 35, 70
fennel   46, 155-6
fiber   22, 84, 103, 107, 125, 145, 147,
156, 159, 172
  extra   97
  high   53, 56, 130, 172
  insoluble   144
  inulin   138
  neutral gentle   22
fiber benefits   144
fiber component   53
fiber/nutrient   50
Filberts/Hazelnuts   100
fish   14, 29, 37, 61, 69-72, 75, 81
  bony   37, 69-70
  raised   71
Fish/Shellfish   79-80
flavonoids   102, 106, 134, 146, 149,
156, 174
Flax   111-12
flora   14, 28-9, 38, 70
  maintaining healthy gut   23
Flounder   37, 70, 79-80
flours   49, 51, 101
Folate   55-6, 62, 83, 100, 109, 119,
126, 131, 142-4, 169
Folic Acid   169
food allergies   9, 11, 13, 17, 23, 25, 29,
153, 174-6
  nut/shellfish   31
food choices   27-8, 31-2
food diary   14, 30
food families   5-6, 9, 11-15, 17-19, 23-
31, 35, 47-9, 53-5, 57, 59-60, 65, 69-73,
75, 81-3, 117-19, 123-5, 131, 141-3,

149-53, 163-5
  alkaline   138, 158
  animal   81
  consumed   153
  key   96
  packed phytonutrient   149
  respective   23
food families analysis   16, 31
food family members   35, 73, 85, 130,
145, 148, 154
food foes   15, 17, 19
food intolerances   9, 11, 64, 174
food log   16-18
food poisoning   69
food sensitivities   2, 8, 10, 175
foods   i-ii, 3, 6-10, 12-14, 16-20, 22-
35, 47-9, 52, 57-8, 62, 64-5, 75-6, 85,
88, 92-3, 111, 115, 160-1, 167-9, 174-6
  alkaline   130, 135
  anti-inflammatory   73, 101, 128, 131
  anti-parasitic   134
  based   109
  best   6
  best clean   34
  brain   103
  consumed   35
  cultured   121
  deficient   167
  dense   114
  documented reactions of   58, 77, 93,
116, 123
  inflammatory   110-11
  ingested   174-5
  low allergenic   130
  offending   10, 18
  packaged   16, 171
  packaged convenience   32
  power   127
  processed   53
  protein source   111
  real   32, 34
formation, protein collagen   168
founding plant member   88
fringe Foodergies   19
fungi   14, 26, 29, 46, 85, 92, 115, 118-

19, 121-4

G

Garlic 40, 128, 163
General Foodergies 124
genes 4, 12, 26, 28, 35
genetics 4, 12-13, 26, 31, 86, 89, 166
Ginger 46, 158, 161, 163
Gliadin 51-2
glutathione 142-3, 145
glutelins 52
gluten 5, 12, 14, 19, 26-7, 32, 52, 54
gluten free 49, 53-4
glycoalkaloids 89, 94, 136, 153, 174-5
Goat 36, 65, 77-8
Goji Berry 45, 88-90
Goose 36, 68, 78
gourds 42, 76, 110, 138
gout 67, 81, 136, 138, 150, 158
grain bread 25
grains 26, 31, 38, 48-9, 51, 53-7, 62,
64, 76, 85, 160, 172
  whole 48, 50
grape 46, 157, 160
grapefruits 45, 153-5, 160
Grass family 48-59, 65, 69, 75-6, 85
114-115, 122, 160
Grouse 36, 68

H

Haddock 37, 79-80
Hake 37, 79-80
Halibut 37, 79-80
ham 36, 67-8
Haricot Beans 39, 82-3
hazelnuts 40, 100, 116-17
health 1-3, 5-7, 14-17, 19-23, 26-9,
31, 33-5, 52, 54, 59, 61, 77, 81, 88, 93-
4, 115-16, 170, 172-4
  best 18, 30, 69
  breast 155, 173
  cardiovascular 136, 144
  compromised 13

eye 156
ill 9, 16, 34
maintaining 32
reproductive 143
visual 167
health benefits 127
  primary 53
Health Coach 17, 30
Health Coaches and Nutritionists 21
healthy eye functions, maintaining
156
heart 2, 91, 99, 110
heat 167-8
hemp 64, 107-9
Herring/Kippers 79-80
hippuric acid 141
histadine 72
hives 9, 11, 16, 29, 35, 53, 72, 96
Honeydew 42, 138-9
hops 41, 107
hormones 65, 143, 170, 172
Horseshoe Crab 79
humans 31, 66-7, 69, 91, 96, 121, 150
hypertension, primary 81

I

Ice Cream 77
IgA 9-11, 175
IgD 9-10, 175
IgE 8-11, 16, 25, 30-1, 96-7, 174-5
IgG 9-11, 49, 166, 175
IgM 9, 11, 175
illnesses 30, 48-9, 60, 89
immune complexes 10
immune reaction 8, 18, 175
immune response 7-8, 10, 15, 52, 96,
174-5
immune system 10, 54, 120, 168, 175
immune system responses 9
immunity 8, 17, 22-3, 26, 168
inflammation 4, 23, 53, 92, 95, 102,
107, 173
inflammatory 55-6, 104-5, 114
intestine 8, 22, 52, 54, 64, 168-9, 172,

174
intolerances 2, 7-10, 12-13, 30, 35, 54,
117, 164, 166, 174-5
  lactose 9, 31, 64, 121
Iodine 73, 170
Iron 56, 65-6, 68, 74, 83, 90, 110,
113, 131, 144, 146, 153, 170, 172

I

jalapeño peppers 89-90
Jasmine 38, 44, 49
Jicama 39, 82-4
juice 8, 13, 21, 141, 154, 162-4

K

kale 29, 41, 132-3, 163
kefir 35, 62-4, 77-8, 118
ketone bodies 169
Kidney Bean 39, 82, 84, 86
kidneys 102, 138, 141, 158, 168
Kiwi 40, 125-6, 160-2
Kohlrabi 41, 163

L

Lamb 36, 65, 79
Latex-Fruit Allergy 126, 135, 146,
160-1
lectins 25, 31, 55, 84, 122, 172-3
leeks 29, 40, 127-8, 163
legumes 9, 39, 55, 62, 82, 84-7, 114-
15, 160, 172
lemon 45, 153-4, 162
Lemongrass 38, 50
Lenthionin 121
Lentil 39, 82-3, 86
Lettuce 42, 137, 160, 163-4
lime 45, 153-4
linolenic acid 108-9, 111
  alpha 108, 173
Lithium 89, 94, 119-20, 127, 131-2,
138, 150, 171
liver 21, 99, 138, 147, 167-9, 172

lobster 38, 72-3, 79, 81, 97
Lox 79
Lutein 56, 91, 129-30
Lycopene 91

M

Maca Root 41, 132-3
Mackerel 37, 70-1, 80
Magnesium 50, 55-6, 83, 100, 103-6,
109-11, 113, 126, 137, 144, 149, 171-2
Maitake 123-4
Manganese 50, 55-6, 74, 83, 98-106,
109-13, 127, 134, 141-2, 144, 147, 150,
157, 171
Mango 40, 128-9, 160-2
MCTs (Medium chain triglycerides)
99
meat 61, 65-9, 78-9 124, 174
medicines 2-4, 28, 49, 52, 65
  commercial 2, 155
Mediterranean diet 148
Menaquinone 168
mental health 52
migraines 12, 117
milk 62, 64, 76-8, 107, 161
  cow's 35, 62-3
  goat's 62
  seed 75, 114
milk proteins 36, 63
milk replacements 62, 64
Millet 38, 50-1, 59
minerals 23, 32, 47, 54, 71, 149, 168,
170-2
mint 43, 76, 112, 160-1
mollusk 73
Monkfish 80
Monounsaturated Fat 98, 101, 105,
173
Mozzarella Cheese 78
mucilage, natural 112-13
Mulberry 44, 145-6
Mullet 37
mushrooms 14, 46, 118-22, 124
mussels 38, 73-4, 79, 81

Mustard Greens 41, 132, 163
Mutton 36, 78-9
Mycoprotein 46
Myrtle 44

N

Naturopath 1-5, 13, 17, 21, 30
Niacin 50, 55, 65, 68, 70, 83, 119, 126, 169
nicotine 20, 91-2, 133
Nightshades 4, 7, 14, 19, 32, 45, 88-9, 92-5
Non-IgE allergic reactions 174
nut allergies 13, 115
nutrition 2, 13
nuts 9, 13, 19, 32, 35, 39, 57, 62, 64, 75-6, 92, 96-108, 114-17, 122, 128-9, 172, 174-5
 avoiding 97
 based 115
 digest 104-5
 edible 100
 hardest 102
 hemp 108
 hickory 43, 102
 macadamia 45, 105
 new-age health 111
 packaged shelled 87
 pine 104, 117
 refrigerate 115
 unique 98
Nuts & Seeds 96, 114, 116

O

oats 38, 49, 51-2, 64, 114
Octopus 38, 79
oils 50, 57, 71, 76, 85, 92, 108, 114, 148, 156
 volatile 156
okra 44, 144-5, 163-4
oleic acid 99-100, 104, 109, 111
Olive 44, 148, 163
Omega-3 55-6, 69, 103-4, 109, 111,

114, 120, 127-9, 134, 136, 140-2, 146-8, 152, 154, 156, 159, 173
 ratio of 84, 135, 139-41
Omega-3 fatty acids 101-2, 114
Omega-6 68-9, 101, 104, 107, 114, 134-6, 139, 141, 144, 146, 148, 156, 173
 higher 109, 111
onion 40, 127-8, 163-4
opiate 52
Oral Allergy Syndrome (OAS) 72, 92, 126, 147, 155, 175-6
oxalates 126, 131, 136, 138, 140, 142, 157
oxalic acid 149-50, 156, 159
oxidation 115, 170
oysters 38, 73-4, 79, 81, 124

P

palmitic acid 99, 109, 111, 174
Paneer 77-8
Papaya 41, 134-5, 160-2
parasites 9, 23, 72, 75
parsley 29, 46, 155-6, 161
parsnip 46, 155-6, 163
peaches 26, 45, 97, 106, 150-1
peanuts 9, 13, 18, 39, 82-6, 99, 115
Pear 45, 151, 160, 162
Peas 39, 82-3
pecans 43, 102-3, 114
Pepitas 110
peppers 45, 89, 91, 93
 hot 7
Perch 37, 80
Persimmon 43, 160, 162
pets 106, 145
Pheasant 36, 68, 78
phospholipids 169-70
Phosphorus 50, 55-6, 62, 65-8, 70, 83, 98, 100, 103-6, 109-13, 144, 168, 171
phytic acid 54, 57, 104, 114
phytonutrients 91, 128-9, 133, 143, 151

Phytosterols 56, 100, 102, 105-6, 109, 134, 139, 142, 154, 156, 159, 173
Pigeon 36
Pike 37, 70, 80
Pine nuts/Pignoli 45
Pineapple 41, 133-4, 160-2
Pinolenic acid 104-5
Pinto Bean 39, 82, 86
Pinyon nuts 104
pistachios 29, 40, 96, 98-9, 116
plant fats 172
plant sterol/stanol esters 53, 98, 109
plant sugars 8
plantain 44, 146-7, 162
Plum 45, 150-1, 160, 162
poisons 7, 174-5
Pollen 58, 76, 85, 93, 160
polyphenols 91, 144, 152-3, 159
Pomegranates 44, 143-4, 162
Poppy Seed 116
Porgy 38, 80
pork 29, 36, 67-9, 76, 81
Potassium 56, 83, 98, 119, 125-6, 132, 135-6, 138, 140, 142, 144, 146-8, 152, 154, 171-2
potato 7, 45, 53, 88-94, 142, 163, 175
  sweet 42, 135-6, 140
poultry 14, 36, 68-9
proanthocyanins 133, 157
probiotics 17, 35, 118-19, 121-2
profile
  complete protein 74, 111, 126
  unique protein 85
prolamines 51-2, 55
properties, sedative 158-9
protease inhibitors 91
pumpkin 42, 110, 138-9, 163-4
Pumpkin Seed 29, 110, 116
punicalagins 144
purines 66-7

Q

quercetin 55, 106-7, 128-9, 133, 141, 174

quinoa 39, 48, 56, 126-7

R

Rabbit 36, 78-9
radicchio 42, 137-8
Radish 41, 132-3, 163
Rancid oils 115
reactions 8-10, 13-15, 17-19, 21-3, 25, 27, 30, 35, 55, 57-9, 72, 76-7, 85, 92-3, 97, 102, 115-16, 123, 141-2, 160-1
  sensitive 57, 76, 85, 93, 115, 123, 160
reactivity, food combination 30
Red Bean 39, 82, 86
reverse ill health 21
rheumatic conditions 67, 126, 136, 138, 158
rhubarb 39, 55, 149-50, 163
Riboflavin 65, 68, 83, 89, 106, 119, 149, 169
rice 38, 48-54, 58-9, 64, 114
Rice Bran 59
Rice Cake/Flour 59
Rice Milk 62, 78
roasted chestnuts 102
romaine 42, 137, 163-4
Rutin 55, 131, 141, 154
Rye 38, 49, 51, 59
Rye Flour 58-9

S

Sailfish 38
salicylates 106, 130, 134, 152, 159
salicylic acid 126, 141-2
Salmon 37, 70-1, 80
Salmonella 69
salt 63, 83, 89, 172
Sardine 37, 70-1, 80
Saturated Fat 100, 104, 106, 173
scallops 38, 73, 79, 81
Sea Bass 37, 70-1
seeds 39, 48-50, 54-5, 57, 62, 76, 92, 96-7, 103, 107-15, 117-18, 122, 129,

146, 152, 154, 172
Selenium   50, 62, 65, 67-8, 70, 72, 74,
90, 103-4, 109, 111, 119, 171
sensitivities   7-9, 11-12, 17, 19-20, 22,
30, 35, 54, 64, 76, 81, 85, 93, 115, 117,
123, 147, 150, 153, 166
sensitivity reaction   57, 76, 134
sesame   45, 113
Sesame Seed   113-14, 116
Shad   37, 80
shellfish   9, 76, 81
shells   97-9, 102, 114-15, 117
Sherbet   77-8
shiitake mushrooms   118-9, 121-4
Shrimp   38, 72-3, 79
skin   9, 15, 17, 21, 23, 29, 52, 89, 94,
130, 135, 139, 142, 147, 155, 157, 168,
175
skin eruptions   9, 11
Snails   38, 73-4, 80
Snipe   36
sodium   67-8, 72-3, 101, 110-11, 114,
148-9, 155-6, 171-2
soil   26-7, 89, 118, 167
solanine   7, 91-2, 127, 138, 141-2, 152,
175
Soluble fibers   172
sorrel   39, 55, 149-50
Sour Cream   78
soy   5, 9, 14, 18-19, 29, 32, 35, 64, 71,
108, 114
soybeans   39, 49, 76, 82-3, 85-6
spinach   38, 56, 126-7, 164
Spirulina   163
Squashes   138-9
Standard American Diet   34, 81, 171
starches   52-3, 115, 122
starchy/carbohydrate   92
starchy vegetables   57, 76, 85, 92, 159-
60
Starfruit   162
sterols   65, 172-3
stimulant, dietary   147
stomach   7-8, 75-6, 85, 92, 115, 122,
128, 159, 174

stone fruits   97, 150-1
Strawberries   45, 150-1
Striped Bass   79
Sturgeon   37, 80
substitute   112-13
sugar beets   38, 50, 56, 126-7
sugars   2, 18, 25-6, 33, 35, 38, 48, 50,
54, 62, 127, 130, 175
sulfur, native   131
Sunfish   37
Sunflower Seed/Butter   116
sunflower seeds   109, 117
sushi   75
symptoms   3, 10-11, 16, 21, 23, 28-9,
49, 72, 107, 121, 176

T

Tahini   116
tannins   55, 98, 101, 130, 138, 144-5,
147, 151, 153, 157
Taro   40
tea   46, 48, 57, 161
Teff   38, 50-1, 58
tests   12, 23, 30, 54, 60, 97
Therbromine   145
Thiamine   50, 56, 66-8, 83, 98, 100,
102-3, 105, 111, 113, 168
throat   97, 176
Tilefish   38, 80
tomato   7, 45, 88-94
tongue   175-6
toxins   ii, 2-4, 13-15, 19, 21-3, 26, 29,
35, 48, 52, 81, 94, 99, 121, 129, 174
trace minerals   89, 108, 170-1
tree   103, 115, 175-6
tree nuts   9
   shelled   86
triglycerides   154, 173-4
Trout   37, 80
True Grasses   38, 48-9
Tuna   37, 70, 80
Turkey   36, 68, 79
Turnip   41, 132, 164

U

UltraSimple Diet   166
Unsaturated fatty acids   109, 111

V

Veal   36, 78
vegan diet landscape   82
vegetables   13, 26, 29, 39, 125, 159-61, 163-4, 175-6
Venison   36, 66, 78-9
Vitamin A   62, 89, 132, 136-8, 147, 153, 155-6, 167, 173
Vitamin B6   147, 169
Vitamin B12   169
Vitamin C   89, 101, 125, 127, 129, 134, 137-8, 140-1, 146, 150, 153, 155, 157, 168, 170-1
  high   83
  source of   83, 89
Vitamin D   4, 6, 72, 92, 119, 121, 168, 170-1
  higher   70
Vitamin D2   168
Vitamin D3   168
Vitamin E   98, 100, 103, 108, 114, 141, 168
Vitamin K   83, 126, 131-2, 142, 144, 150, 153, 155, 168
  high   149
vitamins   23, 32, 47, 50, 54-6, 62, 65-8, 70-3, 83, 98-106, 108-13, 125-7, 129-32, 134, 136-8, 140-4, 146-50, 152-3, 157-9, 167-70

fat soluble   167-8
high   144
missing   33
water soluble   168-70

W

walnuts   43, 96, 102-3, 114, 116-17
water   20, 64, 69, 72, 81, 100, 107, 114, 162, 167, 172
Watermelon   42, 138-9, 160
Western diet   108
Wheat   18, 38, 49-55, 57-9, 101, 161
Wheat Bread   58-9
Wheat Products   9, 58-9
Whey/Whey Protein Supplement   78
White mushrooms   124
Whitefish   37, 70-1
Wild Rice   38, 50-1
winter   17, 139
Wintergreen   40, 43

Y

Yam   43, 135, 140, 163-4
yeast   14, 76, 118-9, 122, 168
Yellowtail   37, 79
yogurt   35, 62, 64, 78, 118

Z

Zinc   50, 55-6, 65-6, 72, 74, 83, 98, 102-4, 106, 109-11, 113, 172

LAURA KEILES ND

ABOUT THE AUTHOR

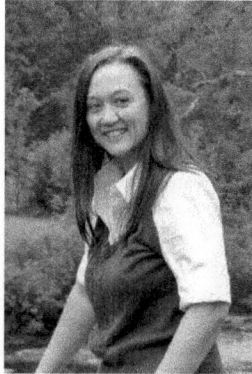

Laura Keiles, PMP, ND, HC is a certified Project Management Professional, Traditional Naturopathic Consultant, Certified Health Coach and certified Gluten Free Practitioner in Hillsborough, NJ. She obtained her certification as a Health Coach from Institute of Integrative Nutrition. She graduated in 2011 with a Doctor of Naturopathy degree from Clayton College of Natural Health. Ms. Keiles has her certification as Project Management Professional since 1995. She has also attended the Integrative Medicine Symposium for Mental Health so that she can find other ways to resolve pain using neuro-psychological supportive remedies. She is Board Certified by American Association of Drugless Practitioners.

In 2008, she was identified with osteoarthritis of unknown origin, and shortly thereafter, with gluten and dairy sensitivity. This became a personal mission to help others learn to live pain free in a pain filled world, as she had learned to. Through a structured project plan of homeopathy, detoxification, cleanses, and dietary modification she found a way to support and maintain her health. She is committed to being the researcher and student, gathering data/information and turning it into knowledge and wisdom to share, and support others on their journey of health improvement.

She live with her husband and two sons and helps them stay healthy and pain-free consuming what ever foods and food families work best for them.

www.ingramcontent.com/pod-product-compliance
Lightning Source LLC
Chambersburg PA
CBHW031157270326
41931CB00006B/305